Living With Chronic Fatigue

Living With Chronic Fatigue

By
Susan Conant

Taylor Publishing Company
Dallas, Texas

Published by Taylor Publishing Company
            1550 West Mockingbird Lane
            Dallas, Texas 75235

Designed by David Timmons

Library of Congress Cataloging-in-Publication Data

Conant, Susan.
    Living with chronic fatigue / by Susan Conant.
        p.   cm.
    Includes bibliographical references.
    ISBN 0-87833-709-1 : $9.95
    1. Chronic fatigue syndrome—Popular works.   I. Title.
    RB150.F37C66   1990
    616.85′28—dc20   89-77048
                                                            CIP

Printed in the United States of America

10 9 8 7 6 5 4

For the people I've called Alex, Alison, Andy, Don, Ellen, Erik, Ginny, Greg, Jean, Kay, Laura, Leah, Marcie, Marian, Marna, Maya, Meg, Mia, Norma, Roseanne, Thalia, and Wendy.

Contents

Introduction

One Saturday morning in October of 1986 I awoke with my eyes even more puffy than I'd learned to expect at forty. I had a low-grade fever. I felt ill, looked ill, and stayed ill. My white blood count went up and down. I developed some joint pain. The fever continued off and on until December of 1987. In searching for a diagnosis and help, I found the medical system to be a second malady almost as bad as the first. In addition to the twin maladies of illness and medicine, I soon discovered a third: other people's well-intentioned misunderstanding. And a fourth: my own despairing confusion.

In search of help for all four ailments, I read whatever I could find, which was very little. Most medical books ignored the existence of unnamed illnesses. What literature I was able to find about chronic Epstein-Barr virus syndrome and chronic fatigue syndrome suggested that if I had CEBV or CFS, I'd probably never recover. What almost everyone offered, in person and in print, was advice: take vitamin C, accept the illness, ignore it, become an exceptional person, reduce the stress in your life, try acupuncture, and find God.

I started this book when I began to recover from my illness. I wanted to write the book I had sought and not found, a book about dilemmas and choices, not symptoms and vitamin supplements.

For diversity of experience and outlook, I turned to twenty-two people, five men and seventeen women, who talked freely and generously with me about themselves and their experiences of illness. One of the women—I call her Thalia—is the healthy mother of an ill child whom I call Marcie. Two other women are a mother-daughter pair; Jean, the mother, is healthy, and Mia, her daughter, is ill. Those are not their real names, nor are the other names I use here. The woman I call Meg had recovered from an acute, life-threatening illness that was nothing like CFS. Andy's illness is, as he says, "this thing," not CFS. Erik may or may not have CFS, CEBV, fibromyalgia, or some form of arthritis. Marian's blood tests show elevated Epstein-Barr virus titers, but she has been unwell off and on for only a few months, and she feels tired rather than ill. I don't know whether she has anything and, if so, what. Maya was initially told that she had CEBV, but I'll save her story for later. Everyone else has or had an illness in the CEBV/CFS family.

Whether your illness has a name or not, you have a chronic fatigue illness if you know that *something* hit you, but neither you nor anyone else knows exactly *what*. This book is about contracting, living with, and recovering from the illness that is now officially called chronic fatigue syndrome. It is also about other illnesses that are not quite officially chronic fatigue syndrome, but are not quite anything else either: fevers of unknown origin, baffling neurological disorders, and illnesses with no name.

Throughout this book I write about "us," "our" illnesses, and what "we" experience. Although I have recovered, in a sense, my illness will always be with me. I find myself unable to write about people who are still unwell as "those people," as if I were distancing myself from them, their illnesses, and their lives.

My purpose in writing this book is to describe the experience of having this strange and baffling illness by exploring issues, dilemmas, myths, and realities. To discover that others also have waxing and waning fevers, swollen glands, exhaustion, joint pain, or other symptoms helps to validate the physical experience of illness. I want to offer whatever support lies in acknowledging some of the equally painful emotional experiences that accompany an effort to define the illness, explain it to other people, find help, and, in the meantime, live with it.

1

Definitions and Diagnoses:

THIS BAFFLING ILLNESS

A universal theme that ran throughout my talks with people who have CFS was the intense frustration of having an illness that defies explanation. Their feelings of bewilderment will be all too familiar to anyone who has or has had a mysterious and long-term ailment.

ROSEANNE: THE "FOREVER FEVER"

"I once climbed Mt. Kilimanjaro," Roseanne tells me, but she hasn't climbed any mountains lately, at least not that kind.

We are talking on the telephone. The phone is her choice. She is too sick to visit me—in fact, so sick and so tired that she no longer drives at all.

"A good day," she says, "it's when I get my own breakfast and lunch. That's a good day." Her tone is matter-of-fact.

Should I have invited myself to her house for our talk? No. I will have to hear her story without seeing her, without meeting her face to face. I remember the exhaustion too well to impose myself on her. My fever lasted only fourteen months. Roseanne has been ill for almost two years.

In April 1987, Roseanne was looking forward to a trip to California. Happily married and the mother of a ten-year-old daughter, she was also an administrative assistant in the graduate school of one of Boston's many universities. She had, as usual, been working hard, but she wasn't tired. After all, this is someone who once climbed Mt. Kilimanjaro.

That April, Roseanne got the flu, or what she thought was the flu. It lasted three weeks. At the end of those three weeks, she had recovered enough so that she and her husband went ahead with their vacation plans; but in California, she says, "I was so fatigued that I could hardly crawl from the hotel room to the pool." After the vacation ended, she was still too ill to return to work. The sick, flu-like feeling, sore throat, swollen glands, and muscle aches still plagued her. At the end of three weeks, she returned to work and cut back her time there to only a few hours a day. But concentration was impossible. She stopped working and spent the next two weeks in bed.

Not until she had been ill for three months did she consult a doctor, and it was Roseanne, not the doctor, who suggested a blood test for EBV, the Epstein-Barr virus. The test results came back, she consulted another doctor, and she was told that she had CEBV, chronic Epstein-Barr virus syndrome. The diagnosis was later amended to CFS, chronic fatigue syndrome. "Now," she says, "they say it's not caused by EBV." Even so, Roseanne sometimes tells people that she has CEBV, a virus. "If I say I have chronic fatigue syndrome, I can hear the dead silence," she says. "I can hear, 'Oh, sure.' If you say *virus*, it's different."

ANDY: "SOME WEIRD THING"

Andy and I talk in his office. He's a psychotherapist with a Ph.D. in clinical psychology. His office is a large, stylishly furnished room in a charming old house. I like the warm light and the comfortable chairs. I like Andy, whom my husband and I have known for years.

Although he's in his early forties, there's no gray in his curly black hair. He looks healthy. His eyes are lively. If I were here for therapy, I realize, I'd find it easy to talk to Andy, but I'm here to listen to Andy's story, not to tell mine.

"I've realized that I'm not in control of my body," he says, "and I'm not my body. I've detached my sense of who I am from this thing that's always in pain."

Four years ago, one of Andy's teeth split, and he eventually had a gold crown put on the tooth. The next morning, he awoke with a headache. After a few days, his dentist evened the crown, but the headache remained. "Then," Andy tells me, "I started getting tingling sensations throughout my body, like novocaine without the numbness. And heat, tremendous heat, like a sunburn. And then it was followed by extreme muscle aches and pains, like arthritic pain." To alleviate these symptoms, Andy takes ibuprofen every three hours, day and night. According to Andy, it makes his life possible.

Unlike Roseanne, Andy doesn't feel sick. "I feel like a very healthy person with some weird thing going on," he says. He does not have chronic fatigue syndrome. What does he have? In the past four years, he's consulted internists, neurologists, and dentists. "Has anyone ever told you that you have MS?" one neurologist asked him, but he doesn't have multiple sclerosis. He's also been told that he has TMJ (temporomandibular joint disorder) and mercury poisoning from the amalgam fillings in his teeth; that he probably has a brain tumor or lupus; and that he definitely has something called marginal sclerosis of the atlantoaxial junction. He's had EEG's, a CAT scan, a brain scan, a spinal series, sinus X-rays, and countless blood tests. Some doctors, psychics, and friends have told him that his pain is psychosomatic.

In addition to the traditional medical and dental routes, Andy has tried what he calls "the alternative world" of acupuncture and chiropractic and "the even more alternative world" of psychics and clairvoyants. He's had all the metal in his teeth replaced with nonmetallic substances. He's worn bite plates in his mouth. Exercise programs, dietary programs, medical clairvoyance, and Rolfing have been no more effective than the more (and less) traditional approaches. "If you're on this journey," Andy asks, "if you're on this path, why not? How is this going to harm me?"

Is this illness, this pain the center of Andy's life? I think not. Many of Andy's friends are my friends, too, and nearly all of them believe that he has recovered. Because I know Andy and his friends, I know that he never, ever talks about the pain. He has never stopped seeing clients and never stopped teaching. A year ago, he married a widow with two teenage children. His new family, not his illness, is the center of his life.

Is he imagining the illness? "I have my doubts sometimes," he says. "I wonder if there is something going on with me, if I'm creating this, but my deepest belief is that I am not doing this to myself." His doctor believes him. Last week, he was back in the hospital for even more tests. Whatever Andy has is not chronic fatigue syndrome, but, so far, neither he nor anyone else has a name for it.

A NAME FOR IT

Chronic fatigue syndrome goes by a variety of names: chronic mono-like illness, chronic Epstein-Barr virus syndrome (CEBV), chronic fatigue and immune dysfunction syndrome (CFIDS), chronic viral syndrome, chronic Epstein-Barr-like syndrome, and post-viral fatigue syndrome.

What about *chronic fatigue syndrome*, the official name approved by the Centers for Disease Control? In her welcoming speech at the San Francisco Chronic Fatigue Syndrome Conference on April 15, 1989, Nancy Walker, a member of the San Francisco Board of Supervisors, said of the term *chronic fatigue syndrome*: "This name really misses the point; it makes about as much sense to me as it would to call diabetes a chronic *thirst* syndrome!"

What's wrong with *fatigue*? First, *chronic fatigue syndrome* suggests continuity with ordinary experience; it sounds like what people have who feel tired all the time. Second, it describes a secondary symptom. The primary sensation, the subjective essence of the illness, is not feeling fatigued, exhausted, or tired, but feeling ill or in pain.

What about the other labels? Why not pick one of the popular ones? Chronic fatigue and immune dysfunction syndrome?

Chronic Epstein-Barr virus syndrome? Both of these labels imply conclusions about the nature of the illness. The immune dysfunction hypothesis is as popular now as the Epstein-Barr hypothesis was a few years ago. I can't pick one of those labels without committing myself to a hypothesis about the nature of the illness, and, when it comes to the cause and nature of the illness, I am an agnostic. Many people, however, are not, and I believe that those people are entitled to the labels they prefer. Consequently, when I am referring to the illness variously called chronic fatigue syndrome, chronic fatigue and immune dysfunction syndrome, and chronic Epstein-Barr virus syndrome, I use any and all of those labels as well as CFS, CFIDS, and CEBV or EBV.

DEFINITION BY EXCLUSION

This book is about living with CFS and other strange chronic illnesses, but it is not about all vague ailments. If you've had a scratchy throat for a week, but your throat culture was negative and your doctor told you that you had some virus, your illness is not CFS. CFS attacks, retreats, ambushes, lays siege, and drops bombs, but it doesn't just quit after a week. Also, this book is about physical illness. If you feel tired, depressed, anxious, confused, or otherwise rotten but you don't have a fever, swollen glands, or some other sign of physical illness—in other words, if you feel lousy but not sick—this book is not for you.

I also want to emphasize that neither this book nor any other will tell you whether you have CFS, CFIDS, or CEBV because they are diagnoses of exclusion: they mean that you are sick but do not have any of hundreds of familiar medical maladies.

KAY: THE SEARCH FOR A DIAGNOSIS

Kay and I sit in the living room of her apartment. It's an attractive room, modern and cheerful, furnished with taste as well as obvious expense. A mid-level executive with a Fortune 500 company, Kay can afford the furniture, the apartment, the good neighborhood. Her appearance fits the apartment. Her curly red hair is styled rather than just cut, and she is wearing a pale dress with chunky jewelry. She looks successful. She does not look ill, except maybe around her eyes, which are circled and a little tired. When we first begin to talk, I sense some distance between us, but once she's heard a summary of my own illness, she evidently trusts me.

Kay's illness began, she tells me, "with neurological symptoms. Numbness. Fine motor coordination. Pretty soon after that, I just started to feel sick. Almost like a flu, but it was getting worse and worse and worse. This was five and a half years ago, so no one had heard of anything called chronic fatigue syndrome." Kay's internist "basically suggested it was stress. He really discounted all the stuff I was telling him about how sick I was feeling. In terms of the neurological stuff, he pretty much discounted that, too." He did, however, refer her to a neurologist "who turned out to be a really wonderful guy, who, among other things, wanted to rule out multiple sclerosis. So that was our operating diagnosis at the time."

The neurologist did rule out MS and "decided after a while that there wasn't anything neurological wrong with me. But he, at least, believed that there was something wrong with me. He just didn't know what it was. He presumed that it was some sort of virus that would eventually run its course and go away. I felt comfortable that everything else was ruled out. I believed that I didn't have MS. I believed that I didn't have cancer. Though it wasn't so much that I believed him as that I didn't know what else to do."

Kay's illness worsened, but "then I sort of got better, quite a bit better, and then I had a relapse." At that point, her neurologist sent her to an infectious disease specialist, who repeated a test for something the neurologist had suspected but that one test had failed to confirm: toxoplasmosis, a parasitic infection. "It was like: Oh, great! A diagnosis! It wasn't a disease that you die from. It was something real. You couldn't do anything about it, but at least it had a name, and that made it less scary."

Kay felt progressively better. Indeed, she felt so much better that she joined a group of friends who invited her to accompany them on a trip to South America. But just before returning home from the trip, she says, "I wasn't feeling well, and I got home, and I still wasn't feeling well. After a while, the symptoms started to feel vaguely familiar. I thought, oh-oh, this is back again. At that point, there was all this stuff about Epstein-Barr in the news. I started to read about it, and I just knew: I have it." Kay consulted her infectious disease specialist, who "tested for the EBV titers—of course, now they know the Epstein-Barr virus isn't necessarily the cause of all this, but at that time they thought it was—and it did happen to be high. (A titer is a measurement of the concentration of a substance in a solution, in this case, antibodies specific to the Epstein-Barr virus.) So then we changed our operating diagnosis to: Well, yeah, you did have toxoplasmosis, but that's not what's making you sick anymore. What's making you sick, the chronic aspect of this, is chronic Epstein-Barr virus. So that started a whole new era."

Kay's route to the diagnosis of EBV, then chronic fatigue syndrome, is in some ways atypical: she rather quickly found a doctor who believed she was ill. That doctor thoroughly and speedily ruled out, to Kay's satisfaction, most of the possibilities she dreaded. Once Kay heard of chronic Epstein-Barr virus syndrome, her doctor immediately tested for the virus and provided the diagnosis. She saw relatively few doctors and few specialists. With the exception of the short time during which her neurologist suspected that she had MS, she did not go through periods of living with a tentative diagnosis of an alarming illness.

FINDING A LABEL

A diagnostic label confers on illness a certain social and personal reality: it announces to the world and to you that you have something that's not just in your head. Nonetheless, a diagnostic label does not necessarily explain anything, especially what caused your problem, nor does it necessarily offer the promise of a cure, nor does it necessarily make the illness predictable. Multiple sclerosis, for example, is a familiar, medically legitimized diagnosis, but the cause of MS is still a mystery.

It seems, however, that a familiar diagnosis at least frees people to stop thinking and worrying about what the problem is and whether it is diagnosable. As author Cheri Register shows in *Living with Chronic Illness* (1987), when people with undiagnosed illnesses desperately long for some familiar label in the hope that the label will somehow help, they are apparently cherishing a well-founded hope. Andy has had numerous diagnoses, each of which has later been discarded. Each time, according to Andy, "It's been wonderfully comforting to have a diagnosis!"

For some people, the label CEBV, CFS, or CFIDS triggers just the kind of relief for which the undiagnosed are looking. Once Don had the CEBV label, he tells me, "I could get a grip on something. I was no longer in the dark." When Leah was finally given that diagnosis, "everything made sense. I realized that I wasn't the only one, and I wasn't crazy." For others, like Marna, the end of the route, the label, is inconclusive and unsatisfying. "I don't think the diagnosis means anything," she tells me flatly.

An unnamed or vaguely named illness often seems to involve a complicated set of conditional uncertainties that feel like a web of guesses, not a reality. CFS, CEBV, and CFIDS can function as psychologically helpful labels. They are increasingly familiar labels that many sick people and concerned doctors are working hard to legitimize. They enable people to say: this is the illness; this is the reality.

A CAUTIONARY TALE

"Did you have arthritis?" I ask Maya.

No, she tells me, just some muscle aches. No fever that she noticed. She didn't have a rash. What she had was fatigue. "Fatigue has so many properties! It was like living with a fifty-pound weight on my limbs. Or like trying to break through a cloud cover. I couldn't get out of bed. I couldn't climb a flight of stairs without sitting down."

Not long after Maya became ill, she found a doctor who had seen many patients with EBV, a doctor who was apparently not surprised to find that Maya's EBV titers were high. She was in many ways the classic EBV/CFS patient. A woman. The right age. "I was working hard, long hours at a high-powered job," she says. Perhaps she, too, was not surprised at the diagnosis. "When you have something like this, you're so relieved to find someone who puts a label on it. I didn't push hard enough to see if it was something else."

The something else was Lyme disease.

The moral of the story is, of course, that chronic fatigue syndrome is not the only cause of the symptoms of chronic fatigue illnesses.

THE RANGE OF DIAGNOSES

To introduce a little order into the confusion of searching for a diagnosis, let's look at some possibilities of what a baffling illness might be.

The Potentially Diagnosable

Your mysterious illness could be a potentially diagnosable disease or disorder, something with a traditional medical label that no one has yet succeeded in matching with your illness. Why might that be?

The problem could be undiagnosed because it is a sneaky sort of thing that lurks around or is just plain hard to diagnose, even for experts. A disorder may produce symptoms that are an unusual way for that disorder to announce its presence.

The illness could be undiagnosed because it is unfamiliar to doctors in your geographic area. The average patient of an American doctor does not have a tropical disease. Obviously, if there is any chance at all that you have a tropical disease, you must consult a specialist in tropical medicine.

Finally, a potentially diagnosable illness or disorder may go undiagnosed because of some kind of medical error, miscommunication, or test inaccuracy. A doctor may miss a diagnosis because of a failure to take a complete medical history, to order crucial tests, or otherwise to do a complete work-up. This is just the kind of failure that doctors and patients fear. The list of typical things any doctor should fear missing is long. It includes hyperthyroidism, toxoplasmosis, cytomegalovirus, Addison's disease, brucellosis, collagen vascular disorders, giardiasis, AIDS, subacute bacterial endocarditis, pneumonia, malignancies, environmental toxins, and many more.

Unfortunately, not all doctors are as thorough as they should be. After she had been working closely with two women who came down with EBV, Alison developed headaches and a sleep disorder. When she began to feel really ill, she went to a doctor who had never seen her before and who did not have her medical records. The purpose of her visit was to ask whether she, too, had EBV. "Sometimes I wish I'd never done it," she tells me as we sit in my living room. She is in her forties, slim, and pretty. There is anger in her voice. "He sent away for the EB titers, and they came back sky high, and he said, 'OK! You have EBV.' My doctor's position was that it was an immune system problem and that if we'd just bolster my immune system, I'd be fine. And I believed that I would." She pauses. "The doctor was really slow to do a complete check-up. He was very supportive, but I kept saying, 'Tell me what's going on chemically.' For instance, I'd had a thyroid problem, so I asked him to check out the thyroid again. But he didn't do a blood test. And I didn't know at the time to push for blood tests of all sorts.

"Then his view was: it's allergies. So he tested me for candida and said, 'Look, you're allergic to wheat. You're allergic to broccoli.' Then he came up with a yeast diagnosis and put me on an anti-yeast medication. It didn't do anything, so he kept putting me on a more narrow diet. And I said, 'What else can you look at? What about my blood? What about my liver?' We had arguments. He'd want to do more acupuncture. He'd give me vitamin C intravenously. And he'd say, 'I think you've got to come back.'"

Alison eventually found her way to a group of doctors at a university hospital. Although her diagnosis is complicated, it includes chronic fatigue syndrome. It also includes a thyroid problem. Of the first doctor, Alison says, "He's a good person. He tried. But he clearly didn't know a lot."

Equivalent Diagnoses

Historians of CFS like to point to outbreaks of mysterious illnesses that include Royal Free disease and Icelandic disease. There is no evidence to indicate whether those or any other mysterious diseases were identical to one another or to CFS. Many people believe that they are. The only contemporary diagnosis that is a strong candidate for the role of a CFS synonym is fibromyalgia.

According to *The Merck Manual of Diagnosis and Therapy* (15th edition, 1987), *fibromyalgia* refers to "a group of common nonarticular rheumatic disorders characterized by pain, tenderness, and stiffness of muscles, areas of tendon insertions, and adjacent soft-tissue structures." The diagnosis offers, first, a name for a collection of unpleasant symptoms and, second, treatment of some kind for the sleep disturbance, aches and pains, and psychological stress that accompany the illness. The treatments appear to be identical to those for CFS.

Systemic Candidosis

Organisms of the *Candida* family, especially *Candida albicans*, are normal inhabitants of our bodies that occasionally cause trouble, producing, as most women know all too well, vaginal infections. In people with leukemia, those who have had organ transplants, those who are receiving certain drugs, and in people with certain other conditions, however, these organisms may cause serious systemic infections.

In *The Yeast Connection* (1987) author William G. Crook argues that those same organisms not only can but often do cause chronic illness in other people as well. When Alison's doctor attributed her illness to candida, he expressed a view of what is variously called systemic candidosis, candidiasis, or moniliasis that diverges radically from the conventional medical view. An article in the February 1987 issue of the *Harvard Medical School Health Letter* reviewing the yeast connection question, concluded, in essence, that there is no connection between the organisms and the wide variety of symptoms that books attribute to them. Perhaps more importantly, the review article issued a strong warning that although some of the recommendations and treatments advocated by yeast-connection proponents are harmless (e.g., avoiding damp places such as cellars where yeasts flourish), others are potentially very dangerous.

Some people with CFS reject the traditional view of systemic candidiasis or include CFS among the conditions that can make candida a serious problem. The chief medical spokesperson for the view that candidiasis plays an important role in CFS is Carol Jessop, M.D. (See her work in issues of the *CFIDS Chronicle*, the official publication of the CFIDS Association.) Whether or not there really is a yeast connection in people with CFS, some people swear that they benefit from harmless anti-yeast practices such as avoiding molds in the environment and following anti-yeast diets.

Dental Diagnoses

Temporomandibular joint (TMJ) disorders are conditions involving the joint at which the jaw meets the skull. There is no question at all that things can indeed go wrong with this joint. There is now, however, a vogue for attributing to TMJ disorders a variety of both vague and specific symptoms. As with the yeast connection, the main problem with the jaw connection theory is treatment. In this case, one treatment consists of uncomfortable, unpleasant, and expensive oral surgery. TMJ is one of the many diagnoses Andy has had. "One of the dentists suggested it was TMJ," he tells me with more good cheer than I'd have been able to voice, "so I embarked on a couple of thousand dollars' worth of occlusion and bite plate work. But, guess what? That wasn't the problem."

A second dental diagnosis in vogue is chronic poisoning from material used in fillings, especially amalgam, an alloy of mercury and silver. Amalgam fillings contain mercury, and mercury can indeed cause poisoning. The debate is about whether the amount of mercury in fillings is sufficient to cause symptoms of poisoning, or sufficient to cause those symptoms in some especially susceptible people. Andy, open to almost any possibility, had all of his fillings replaced. "I had all the metal removed from my head," he tells me. "Gold, silver, anything. And an intravenous vitamin C flush. And a six-month nutrition program to help remove mercury. It was a wonderful program. Didn't change a thing, but I liked the people a lot."

If dentistry were free and painless, the tentative diagnosis of mercury poisoning from amalgam fillings would be well worth pursuing for anyone with symptoms potentially attributable to mercury. Before packing your life savings into your teeth, however, you should at least read up on the latest reputable research on this diagnosis.

Viruses

As-yet-unrecognized viruses constitute such an important group of potential culprits in baffling illness that they deserve special attention.

One popular view is that CFS/EBV/CFIDS is caused by one particular but as yet unidentified virus. The popular term CEBV reflects a hypothesis about which virus is the culprit: the Epstein-Barr virus (EBV), which causes mononucleosis. Research has shown that although the Epstein-Barr virus may indeed be the culprit in some cases, there is no consistent association between the syndrome and the virus. Some theories state that the illness reactivates viruses, including the Epstein-Barr virus. According to an article in the July 1988 issue of the *Harvard Medical School Health Letter*, "what has emerged from research done so far on chronic fatigue is the general conclusion that neither EBV nor any other common virus is the sole cause of this disease."

Immune Dysfunction

CFIDS, chronic fatigue and immune dysfunction syndrome, it's sometimes called. Some of us get sick, while others living almost identical lives in identical contexts stay well even after they've kissed us. Why? Something has gone wrong in our immune systems. What? Something innate. Or acquired. The result? The dysfunction is making us sick. Or vulnerable to viral infections. It sounds plausible. But it is still just a theory.

Unknown Causes

Odd allergies? Hypersensitivity to substances in the environment that don't bother other people? Unidentified organisms? Dysfunctions in systems other than the immune system? Genetically determined vulnerability to viruses, allergens, or something else? They haven't been ruled out.

What Is a Syndrome?

A syndrome is a group of things that occur together, and, in particular, the symptoms and signs typical of a disease, disorder, or illness. That clarity of particular symptoms and the agreement that the symptoms co-occur is often missing from chronic fatigue syndrome. Roseanne and Don, among others, give almost identical descriptions of their symptoms. Both report muscle aches, swollen glands, and a sore throat. Both use the word "flulike." Marna, with the same diagnosis, describes "a constant cold," wheezing, a fever, and muscle aches. Her most troublesome symptom has been extreme dizziness. Marna describes what she calls distinct "episodes" of illness, not a perpetual, if waxing and waning, flulike feeling. Greg, too, reports that he has "bouts," but in dramatic contrast to Roseanne, Alison, and others who say that they had always been notably strong and robust, he says, "I don't know that I ever knew what it was to feel normal. I know at least a dozen people who say it's been lifelong."

Many illnesses have typical, common symptoms. The same microorganism may, however, manifest itself in different ways in different people, and some of those people may not only feel but objectively be much sicker than others. The syndromic question about chronic fatigue, then, is really a series of questions. Are there, in fact, typical, common symptoms that co-occur, thus defining one clinical syndrome? Or, are there a variety of different syndromes or sub-syndromes? On the basis of a rough look at reported symptoms, it would seem that Roseanne and Don have the same thing, and that Marna has something quite different. If so, are there potentially identifiable viruses associated with the different syndromes? Is there no syndrome at all, but simply two symptoms, malaise and exhaustion, that many people have in common? Is there one offending microorganism, environmental irritant, or immune dysfunction that is making many people feel ill in a variety of bewilderingly different ways? If so, is it a virus? If so, which one? An immune dysfunction? What kind? "I don't believe it's one disease process," says Norma. Greg is convinced that we all have the same thing.

YOU MAY NOT GET A DIAGNOSIS

Suppose you have no diagnosis. The unhappy fact is that not everything is diagnosable. In the absence of a diagnosis, too, the diagnostic possibilities are multiple and complex. When you are first sick, you probably don't even know the names for most of the things you might have. Even after you learn the labels, you are apt to have the sense that you have no idea what's going on. It is also very difficult to evaluate how possible or realistic some of the apparent possibilities are. Once you start to entertain some of the improbable possibilities, you may start to wonder whether your ability to differentiate between fantasy and reality has gone the way of your health.

If you have a diagnosis of chronic fatigue syndrome, CEBV, CFIDS, chronic viral illness, or whatever, the diagnosis is apt to be just about as uncertain as the illness itself. One doctor tells you that you probably have CEBV. Your blood, however, shows that your Epstein-Barr antibodies look just the way you'd expect them to look in someone who had mononucleosis 20 years ago. You then read an article that says that the Epstein-Barr virus has little or nothing to do with your kind of chronic fatigue and fever. Besides, according to another article, people with CEBV have muscular weakness that you don't have. But you also saw a list of sixty-four possible symptoms of the syndrome, and if that list is accurate, you fit the picture. Is there just one syndrome? If so, do you have it? If not, is there anyone else in the world who has your illness, or are you some kind of medical freak?

You may begin to suspect that whatever baffling diagnosis you were given might have little to do with your symptoms, which acquire, by contrast, an almost comforting sort of reality. They are definite. If you have chronic neck pain and headaches and you meet someone else without those symptoms but with a chronic fever, swollen glands, and the same baffling diagnosis as yours, you may well wonder. The diagnosis might, for instance, be a function of the particular doctor who diagnosed you.

ERIK: ALLERGIC "TO EVERYTHING"

When people ask Erik what he has, he says: "Superallergies. I'm allergic to myself." What does he have? One morning three years ago, when he was 25 years old, he awakened feeling unwell, with stiffness and soreness in his joints, especially his knees and hips. "For six months," he says, "I toughed it out. This was the first time I'd ever been sick, and I didn't believe in going to doctors." He eventually consulted a rheumatologist, who identified his illness as fibromyalgia. Another doctor tested him for EBV, however, and told him that he had CFS and that fibromyalgia was not an issue. Another said that the EB virus may have caused the fibromyalgia. Another said frankly that he didn't know, but suspected a postviral problem. When Erik complained of a lump in his throat, he was first told that his symptom signified nothing more than hysteria. The doctors at a famous clinic disagreed: they immediately tested for and found a thyroid problem. Treatment for the thyroid problem, however, did not end the illness; and although an allergist recognized Erik's multiple allergies, the treatment of those has not ended the illness either. Erik's diagnoses depended on which doctor he visited, and in the end, no one was certain. "There's a real question," says Erik, "if I have or had CFS."

THE EFFECT OF SEARCHING FOR A DIAGNOSIS

Regardless of the label and the concept, you lack a cure. You also lack the expectations, however uncertain they may be, that normally accompany an illness. You do not know whether the illness is permanent or temporary; or whether, if it is temporary, when it will leave. You have no way to distinguish between what is and is not a symptom of your illness. A headache could be just an ordinary headache, or it could be a new symptom that will last indefinitely. It could be an incurable symptom with which you will have to live, or it could be the key to a definite diagnosis of something familiar and curable. You may also encounter one of the central dilemmas of uncertain illness: the active search for a clear, specific, verifiable diagnosis undermines adaptation to the illness; and adaptation to life with the illness undermines the pressure to search actively for a diagnosis and hence undermines the chance of finding real help, however small that chance may be. It is difficult to decide whether the wiser course is to adapt to the illness or to struggle for a clear explanation and possible help. If you are not satisfied with the label CEBV, CFS, or CFIDS, you feel confused as well as sick. And often, living with the uncertainty can be as painful as living with the illness itself.

2

Waiting Rooms and Skepticism:

DEALING WITH THE MEDICAL COMMUNITY

When Leah became ill, she belonged to a health maintenance organization (HMO) where she had had the same primary care physician for twelve years. After a long series of misdiagnoses and unproductive consultations with specialists within the organization, she made an appointment with an infectious disease specialist outside the HMO. Her primary care physician at first refused to authorize the referral. Although he finally agreed to do so, the HMO refused to pay for any laboratory tests outside its own facilities. Leah consulted the infectious disease specialist. His laboratory drew blood for EBV tests and sent it to the HMO's laboratory, where it was promptly lost. Having kept some of the blood, the specialist had the test performed. The results showed high EBV titers, and the specialist told Leah, "Look. The clinical picture is of this illness. The titer alone doesn't mean anything, but you have the full clinical picture, and this is what you have."

To Leah's surprise, her primary care physician at the HMO seemed to take neither the diagnosis nor her illness seriously. "So," she says, "I decided I wanted to be transferred. He didn't listen to me. This person had been my doctor for twelve years, and I had total trust in him. I had chosen him because he was health oriented! I didn't understand that he was health oriented because he couldn't tolerate sickness. It wasn't until I got sick that I realized: I've made a relationship with the wrong person."

INSTANT DIAGNOSIS AND DISBELIEF

According to the July 1988 issue of the *Harvard Medical School Health Letter*:

> The current popularity of chronic fatigue syndrome as a diagnosis has created the hazard that both doctors and their patients will too hastily assume that fatigue is a result of this syndrome and neglect to look for other treatable causes. On the other hand, there appear to be people with a real illness that can be called chronic fatigue syndrome; they may suffer not only from their symptoms but from lack of appropriate sympathy for their situation.

There are doctors who issue the diagnosis of chronic fatigue syndrome without eliminating all other possibilities or even the probable ones; there are others who, refusing to believe in the existence of chronic fatigue illnesses, refuse to believe that the patient is sick.

Maya met those in both categories. The infected tick from which she contracted Lyme disease must have bitten her in August of 1988. Although the first major criterion of the CDC (Centers for Disease Control) case definition of chronic fatigue syndrome, published the previous March in the *Annals of Internal Medicine*, states that the fatigue must have lasted at least six months, and although the same article points out that there is no evidence of a causal relationship between the Epstein-Barr virus and the syndrome of chronic fatigue, Maya was told in September that she had chronic Epstein-Barr virus syndrome. According to the article:

> With the apparent lack of correlation between serum Epstein-Barr virus titers and the presence of chronic fatigue symptoms, it is premature to focus research and diagnostic efforts on

Epstein-Barr virus alone. Many public health officials and clinicians are concerned that a diagnosis of the chronic Epstein-Barr virus syndrome may not be appropriate for persons with chronic fatigue who have positive Epstein-Barr virus serologic tests, and that definable occult diseases may actually be the cause of symptoms such as fatigue, weakness, and fever.

Throughout that fall after the article's appearance, Maya paid $250 each month for EBV serologic tests. In addition to consulting EBV experts, she saw a doctor who did not believe she was ill at all. He kept her waiting for half an hour, did almost no tests, and performed an exam she describes as "cursory."

"We see lots of women who have problems at work," he told her. "This is just a reaction to stress. Go back to work."

"Oh, you mean that Epstein-Barr thing?" a doctor asked Mia. "That doesn't even exist."

COMMUNICATION PROBLEMS

Doctors are supposed to be able to diagnose illness and they are supposed to be able to help. The doctor confronted with a patient whose illness resists a diagnosis that can be confirmed by tests is thus a frustrated, failing doctor, inevitably not at his best.

Furthermore, in the effort to find a solid, well-recognized diagnosis, the doctor must refer the patient for tests and consultations, and the doctor cannot control the patient's experiences in those situations. As the number of consultants you see and the number of tests you have increase, so does the probability of a bad experience.

The popular explanation for most of those bad experiences is poor communication between doctor and patient. Poor communication, including the patient's sense of not being heard, is not limited to comparatively mild illnesses with symptoms easily dismissed as imaginary. At the age of thirty-seven, after numerous ovarian cysts and bouts with endometriosis, Meg and her gynecologist decided that she should have a hysterectomy. Immediately after the surgery, Meg developed intense pain; then her liver and spleen became enlarged, and abnormalities appeared in her blood. After consultations with many specialists, three hospitalizations, and numerous tests, she remained acutely ill, and no one doubted that her undiagnosed illness was a serious, perhaps life-threatening one. Meg had an unusually good relationship with her own doctor. Nonetheless, she said exactly what I heard from many people with chronic fatigue syndrome: "I learned that doctors don't listen."

Research generally confirms that doctors and patients communicate little and badly. The doctor, having gone to medical school, must have trouble figuring out just what knowledge to assume you have, lack, need, want, and will or won't grasp. "We are testing you for Addison's disease" may scare the patient who thinks, "Help! I have something so awful I've never heard of it," but reassure the patient who thinks, "Oh, John Kennedy had that."

Feeling sick also brings out the communicative worst in most people. When you mainly want to complain that you feel awful and to plead for help, it is difficult to organize information and state it clearly. It is difficult to know what information the doctor will find relevant and irrelevant. When you have been sick for a long time, the whole situation becomes almost impossible. By then, you've thought of hundreds of things that might hold the key to the illness. Your great-aunt, with whom you once spent an hour twenty-five years ago, had tuberculosis; you once visited the Dominican Republic; you have a spot on your left forearm. If you are seeing a new consultant, you have little idea about what she already knows and wants to know. By then, too, you are apt to be so caught between the anger at still being sick and the hope that this doctor will be one who will help that words fail you. Not all bad experiences, however, are attributed to poor communication. Among the most common sources of frustration with the medical system is the sense that diagnostic efforts are maddeningly slow and that you are forced to wait and wait while medicine drags its heels.

RATIONALIZATIONS

Two good ideas are popular rationalizations for heel dragging. The first is cost containment. It is clearly a good idea not to waste money on unnecessary tests. If you really do have endocarditis, there is no point in wasting money on tests for anything else. The second is patient protection. Since some medical tests pose risks to the patient, the smaller the number of tests, the lower the risk.

If you belong to a health maintenance organization, you may be certain that no one will ask for your opinion about cost containment: minimizing costs is how health maintenance organizations make money. And your doctor cannot change the policies of the HMO; it is her employer. Only after you get sick do you realize that there was a good reason why what you joined was called a health plan: it wasn't an illness plan.

DEFENSIVE MEDICINE

The increasing need for doctors to protect themselves against malpractice actions gives them little leeway to minimize long-term risk and short-term discomfort. From the patient's point of view, it is difficult to tell whether you are being spared, whether you are the victim of cost containment, or whether the doctor is practicing defensive medicine.

In recent years, the threat of malpractice action has increased so greatly that doctors really need to protect themselves. The increase in the popularity of malpractice actions has eroded the best protection against defensive medicine and malpractice action itself: a good relationship between the doctor and patient. The need for defensive medicine does not mean that you speedily receive tests likely to result in a diagnosis; on the contrary, it means that money must be spent on tests possibly irrelevant to your illness that are necessary to protect the doctor.

When Don's illness, subsequently diagnosed as EBV/CFS, started, he had been a member of a health maintenance organization for five years. A year later, his doctor concluded that Don had a viral illness. Don did not find the description helpful. "It was hellish," he says. "I didn't know what was wrong." At some point in the second year of the illness, he asked for a second opinion and was referred to another of the HMO's internists, who, after a battery of tests, said that the illness was "functional, i.e., psychosomatic," Don says. The internist referred Don to the HMO's mental health department, where he saw a psychiatrist whom he found unhelpful. The next week, Don developed pneumonia.

AMBIGUOUS TEST RESULTS

That kind of experience is much less common than something that is a problem for doctors and patients alike: the ambiguity of test results. Many tests are subject to error, and even tests with low error rates may give results that are difficult to interpret. People with active tuberculosis can show a negative response to a tuberculin skin test. A positive response to a second strength tuberculin test can mean that your body is reacting to having a lot of stuff injected, not that it is responding to the tuberculin. Maya's first test for Lyme disease gave a negative result because it was given too soon after she had become infected.

NO DIAGNOSIS, NO TREATMENT

One of the most fundamental principles of contemporary American medicine is that treatment should always be directed to the cause of symptoms. Doctors define themselves as practicing good medicine when they proceed from symptoms to precise diagnosis to treatment based on that diagnosis. Treatment on the basis of symptoms and in the absence of diagnosis is frowned upon for two practical reasons. First, the wrong treatment might make the patient sicker. Second, the wrong treatment might make diagnosis difficult or impossible. If a person with an internal abscess is pumped full of some broad spectrum antibiotic, the antibiotic may fail to clear up the abscess but get rid of the bacteria in the bloodstream so that they can't be identified.

It is, of course, sometimes necessary to treat patients before reaching a precise diagnosis or before identifying the microorganisms responsible for an illness. Laboratory tests, especially blood cultures, are not speedy, and doctors sometimes have to start patients on antibiotics before the results of cultures are available. Doctors must sometimes make educated guesses to prevent patients from dying. But, doctors don't like that. And if they don't like that, you know how happy they are to take guesses about patients who are only mildly or moderately unwell.

BLACKBALLING

"I think you should see someone else," said Ginny's doctor in referring her to their HMO's mental health department. "I felt blackballed," Ginny says. A referral to a mental health department or another source of psychotherapy could, of course, signal the doctor's recognition that a chronic fatigue illness is too difficult to bear alone, a recognition that you need someone on your side who will listen and help. In practice, it seldom means that, and within health maintenance organizations, it sometimes means just what Ginny understood it to mean: you have been blackballed. Medical services for your illness are now cut off.

YOUR DOCTOR VISITS

Illness brings out the worst in us. A visit to the doctor may bring out the worst of the worst. If you have a chronic fatigue illness, you should expect to be often discouraged, tired, depressed, frightened, or angry. Some of us remain coldly controlled. Some of us cry. Some of us remain coldly controlled until we burst into tears. We feel ashamed of ourselves. Some of us act charming. We all feel sick.

Responses to Difficulty

The communicative worst that a chronic fatigue illness brings out in us is not limited to our difficulty in expressing ourselves. We also have trouble understanding what is said to us by doctors. The field of medicine has so many technical terms that a healthy layperson often finds it difficult to follow an explanation, let alone a person who feels sick and exhausted.

One response to difficulty in dealing with the doctor is to seek information elsewhere. Many people with chronic fatigue study up on anything and everything that could possibly be causing the illness.

A friend of mine who has Epstein-Barr keeps a dictionary of medical terms and a copy of *The Merck Manual of Diagnosis and Therapy* next to her telephone. A person with a chronic fatigue illness who picks up *Time* automatically looks for the Medicine section. People read encyclopedias, newsletters of self-help organizations, popular guides to family health, books about medical detection, and *The New England Journal of Medicine*; watch medical shows on television; and attend lectures on chronic fatigue syndrome.

People with chronic fatigue illnesses not only read these things but photocopy and distribute the good parts to fellow sufferers. Many people with a chronic fatigue illness soon accumulate many file folders of newspaper and magazine clippings, reprints from medical journals, and photocopied pages of medical books. People not only read but re-read and study this material until some of it is committed to memory.

"I read a lot about sickness," Leah tells me. I can see that she is someone who reads a lot; her office is lined with books. "I sent away for all those dreadful articles, those dreadful medical articles. I read the *Merck Manual*. I mostly turned to those articles that looked like they might give me information with which to manage my own illness. I was like a person who combs the beach with a coin finder, a metal detector. It was like I had a detector: what can help *me?*" Andy, too, uses Leah's metal-detection approach. Told that he probably had lupus, he checked out books on lupus from the public library; told that had probably had MS, he obtained material from a multiple sclerosis society. He reads up on each tentative diagnosis. I became so obsessed with TB that I once actually read in its entirety a long, detailed book about the blood of tuberculosis patients. It didn't have much of a plot.

Having thus devoted hours, days, and weeks to research on chronic fatigue illnesses, some people deluge their doctors with photocopies of the entire contents of all of the rapidly expanding file folders. Others, and I fall in this category, not only say nothing to the doctor about doing all of this reading but practically disguise the fact that they are doing it. Why? Some patients find that their doctors react negatively to their efforts to learn about CFS. For a long time, Ginny says, she made the mistake of revealing medical knowledge and vocabulary gained in her work to the doctors at her HMO. "But," she says, "once I went in and acted as if I knew *nothing*, things went better." Also, there is something presumptuous about our own unskilled research. As Alison said, "I'm furious at myself for believing I could think my way out of it. I really took it upon myself to figure it out, because I felt that the doctors didn't know what they were doing." To the extent that we are trying to diagnose or explain our illnesses, we are taking upon ourselves a task for which we are untrained. We have, however, pathetically high motivation: the desperate wish to find out what is wrong with us and to recover from it.

This motivation means that CFS patients often know more about the very latest research than doctors themselves do. A new, fast, accurate test for Lyme disease? The hypothesis that CFS is caused by a retrovirus? Dr. Peterson's trials of ampligen with CFS patients? Jean knows about them because she reads everything published about CFS. If she wants to know about experimental treatments for her daughter, Mia, who has been ill for six years, Jean gets on the telephone and finds out. Does the average medical practitioner follow the CFS literature as closely as Jean does? Probably not, unless he is a CFS specialist.

The Need for Active Effort

For the doctor, a diagnostic effort is useless if it yields no new information. For the patient with no diagnosis, however, a diagnostic effort may be psychologically therapeutic. For doctors, diagnostic efforts have only one point: to diagnose the illness. For patients, however, diagnostic efforts serve an additional function: they demonstrate an active effort to help. If someone has bothered to take a sample of your blood and to look at it, then someone is at least trying. Someone cares. People have not entirely given up on you. There were many times when I clung to the knowledge that in some laboratory somewhere, a small, although probably futile, effort was being made to help me.

The sense that avenues of potential help are being ignored is, of course, maddening. Meg, hospitalized with an acute, undiagnosed illness, heard about a new computer program developed at the same hospital in which she was staying. Perhaps because she works with computers, the idea of the program appealed to her; she understood the computer's ability to systematically examine all possibilities. Her doctors, however, refused to try the program. "It was like a blow to the doctors' egos," she says.

Ginny applied to see a famous infectious disease specialist who devotes his research and clinical practice to chronic fatigue syndrome. She filled out and returned the questionnaire sent by his office. Eight months later, she was offered an appointment. Although her regular doctor "kind of went along," she received "zero cooperation" from others at her HMO. "I requested to have my records sent, and they sent half, and not the most recent half either." The HMO eventually paid for that consultation, but it took Ginny a year to have the payment authorized.

Are requests and demands, in fact, unreasonable once the diagnosis of a chronic viral illness, CFS, or something similar has been made? "Once they think they've diagnosed it, they tend not to be vigilant," says Maya, who is still recovering from what turned out to be Lyme disease.

"If I meet a doctor at a party, I get defensive," Mia says. "You can hear it in my voice." Almost anyone with a chronic fatigue illness at some point responds defensively to bad experiences with doctors. One doctor needlessly dwells on the fact that you may never recover. Another contradicts himself and confuses you. Almost everyone makes you wait. Many don't believe that you're ill. Often, doctors seem as baffled by CFS as their patients are. You are scared and discouraged, but saying so elicits no help. You may start out with an attitude of openness and trust, but you often end up feeling angry, fearful, suspicious, and skeptical. Then there is the insult of not being believed. "Go back to work!" we are told. "You look perfectly healthy to me."

False Composure

When you have to see a doctor, one option is, of course, to present the doctor with the raw truth of how hurt, frightened, miserable, angry, and otherwise vulnerable you really are. As Roseanne tells

Susan Conant

me, "You feel so ill, you can't imagine you're not dying. You forget what you were before." Another option is to enter the doctor's office with all of your socially offensive defenses on maximum alert. You go to pieces or you act nasty. There must be some way to save face, and there is: you pull yourself together, reveal none of your feelings, display impeccably polite behavior, and maintain perfect composure.

Presenting such a facade of composure takes a terrible amount of energy and time. I used to have to dress for the part. I would take a shower, put on makeup, fix my hair, and dress carefully. I breathed slowly and deeply. I must certainly have seemed tense, but I didn't seem vulnerable and I didn't seem like a neurotic wreck. False composure represents an effort to save face, but it represents an adaptive effort in another important way, too: if you successfully avoid presenting the doctor with all of the distracting emotional junk attached to the illness, maybe the doctor will be able to focus exclusively on the medical problem, not blame you for it, and figure out how to help.

It sounds like a good idea, but it doesn't work too well. If you really succeed in pulling yourself together, and, in particular, if you look fairly good, you convey the message that you need much less help than you really do. Instead of zeroing in on your medical problems, the doctor may conclude either that you're a healthy hypochondriac or that you are learning to live with your illness so nicely that there is no need for the vigorous effort you would like.

I also found that the emotional price of false composure was high. Acting composed is very exhausting, and it may be followed by the further exhaustion of falling completely to pieces the minute you leave the doctor's office. Particularly discouraging is a vivid sense of being in a no-win situation: if you fall apart, you invite attention to your need to adapt to the illness. If you let your frustration, anger, and hostility show, you invite blame for your illness and a lot of advice about stress. If you act calm, dignified, polite, and pleasant, you may leave the doctor's office just as unhelped as when you entered. If this situation has left you feeling trapped and discouraged, you are not alone; many CFS patients report feeling exactly the same way.

LIVING WITH CHRONIC FATIGUE

Confusion

Alison, whose CFS is complicated by a thyroid problem and traumatic injuries, says of chronic fatigue syndrome, "It has this huge array of symptoms. There's no diagnosis. There's no treatment. I mean, there's nothing." You are tested for something three times, and the results are negative. You conclude that you don't have it. When the test is done yet a fourth time, you start to wonder: I thought I didn't have that, but now maybe I do; so maybe I could really have any of the things I thought were ruled out.

Maybe you're also reading a lot of medical books and articles that you don't entirely understand. The ones you do understand contradict one another. Almost all possibilities seem open, and the strength of your need to know what's going on muddles your thinking still further. "You get so desperate, you can't tell whether you're spending millions chasing straws," Maya says. To your old symptoms you add a new one: a mild thought disorder. I was often simply unable to think straight about my illness.

Deceit

After I had been sick for about nine months, I was feeling pretty desperate. I had recently seen my doctor, who had no help to offer. At that point, I noticed in our medicine cabinet some penicillin that had been prescribed for my husband by his dentist. My husband no longer needed the penicillin, and the little bottle had a sticker with the magic word: refillable. I refilled the prescription, took the penicillin, and stayed sick. Everyone else had given up, but I, at least, was still trying. Did I tell my doctor what I was doing? Not on your life.

My little deceit was unusual, partly, I think, because most doctors are somewhat more willing than mine were to try antibiotics and partly because most patients lose faith in conventional medicine more quickly than I did. There are people with CFS taking experimental drugs brought into the U.S. from Mexico, Canada, and Israel; the network that supplies drugs without FDA (Food and Drug Administration) approval to people with AIDS supplies people with CFS as well.

Furthermore, some who seek alternative help find themselves practicing a deceit similar to mine. After four years of an undiagnosed illness, Andy is an expert on alternative treatments. "I've been to many different health practitioners," he tells me. "What happens with a client like me is that people are threatened by other people's work. You may be seeing a person in one profession and also someone in another profession who doesn't approve of the first. I find that I have to keep quiet when I'm dealing with certain medical people about seeing alternative people. With alternative people, too, I feel like I have to hide from them that I'm getting CAT scans and EEG's."

The Need to Pester

To pester a doctor means, I think, to make multiple annoying demands; for instance, to call repeatedly, to leave messages asking to have your calls returned, and to make requests that have already been met or turned down. I have reluctantly concluded that if you have a chronic fatigue illness, one, and sometimes the only, alternative to pestering is being ignored. Doctors may often be unaware of the experiences that have driven an otherwise nice, polite person to become a pest.

After Ginny's doctor lost a set of test results for two months, she made appropriate adaptations. For subsequent tests, "I hounded them for results." She adds: "It became clear that I wasn't wanted. I don't enjoy making a nuisance of myself."

People who have been ill for many years, however, often sound like Alison, who says, "Now I go in for check-ups, but I try to set more and more distance between visits to doctors because there isn't anything they can do at this point."

Why Doctor Visits Can Be Frightening

Efforts to diagnose a mysterious illness include, of course, tests for disorders of which everyone is afraid, and the testing elicits fear. The results of one test sometimes raise the possibility of a frightening disorder that cannot be ruled out until a second test is done; and the time spent waiting for that second test and then waiting for the result is simply horrible. Ginny spent a week believing that she might have tuberculosis of the kidneys. A gallium scan revealed "something" in my liver. To find out what, I waited for an ultrasound and then waited for the results of the ultrasound. Wendy was told that she had lupus. Others have heard that they may have MS, brain tumors, or AIDS. Encountering a doctor may mean confronting the perplexing, confusing, maddening nature of the illness. This means doctor visits are often one of the worst things about the illness.

Hostility Toward Doctors

To have chronic fatigue syndrome or another baffling illness is in some ways to find yourself a child in a world without grown-ups, a sinister world in which illness erupts as control vanishes. You have the power to control neither the illness nor the diagnostic effort nor the behavior of the doctors you see nor the consequences of the illness for your life. When the reality is that no one has any idea what is making you sick or what to do about it, it is very easy to believe that someone does but won't tell you: better to have this illness become a world with bad adults than a world with none at all. Doctors become those adults, the Mommy and Daddy who could help but don't care. Rage at the illness then becomes rage at the doctor, and the doctor comes to personify the illness.

Is It the Doctor's Fault?

"Treat the patient and not the disease" should not mean: "Treat the patient instead of the disease." But if the patient has a genuinely mysterious illness, the doctor has no choice. "I realized medicine wasn't as advanced as I thought," Maya says. If the illness is not treatable, then the poor doctor has nothing to treat except the patient, and, by that time, many of us are ungrateful patients indeed.

Good News—There Are Exceptions

If you have a chronic fatigue illness, you learn to expect from the health care system every problem you've ever had with it and a few new ones. Sometimes you are happily surprised. I really like my doctor. She is a kind, good human being who knows a lot about medicine and does not tell sick people to have nice weekends.

Of her general practitioner, Meg says unabashedly, "I love him." Throughout her acute illness, "He'd call me, and we'd talk for hours. He was my savior." For those with chronic fatigue syndrome, the savior may be the first doctor who makes the diagnosis and who validates the person's experience of having a physical illness. Of the expert who diagnosed what was then called chronic active Epstein-Barr virus syndrome, Ellen tells me, "He was my lifeline, the only one who understood." For others, the diagnosis does not necessarily entail understanding. Roseanne, for example, was diagnosed with EBV when she had been sick for about three months, but, she says, "It took a year to find a doctor who understood the illness. It's made a world of difference, psychologically. He's got me convinced I'll fully recover. He believes it's a real illness, that it's not psychosomatic. He trusts me."

Making It Work

Roseanne is not ungrateful. Of her doctor, she says, "He practices the *art* of medicine, not the *science* of medicine." Meg calls her doctor "my savior." Alex tells me that he and his doctor "have joined forces and hung in there together." Long before the Epstein-Barr virus hit the news, Laura's family practitioner hit the medical journals and presented her with photocopies of articles on chronic mononucleosis and CEBV; and it was her doctor, not Laura, who initiated many active diagnostic efforts to find another, familiar diagnosis for her illness. When Greg refers to himself and his doctor, he always says "we."

You might not find the perfect doctor, even after a lengthy search. But understanding the medical community (especially their own frustration with a disease that defies diagnosis) and knowing what to expect from a doctor visit should at least make dealing with health-care professionals a better experience than it otherwise might be.

3

Fighters and Malingerers:

IMAGES OF OURSELVES

Stealthy Epidemic of Exhaustion: Doctors Are Perplexed by the Mysterious 'Yuppie Disease,'" announced a June 29, 1987, *Time* magazine article. Yuppie Fever, Yuppie Flu, Yuppie disease, it's called. Who are we, those who get this maligned and stylish plague? Materialistic overachievers who get what we deserve? Our culture offers a number of images of the sick person, including a subset of images about the person with a chronic fatigue illness. The images reside out there in books, films, television shows, and other people's minds; in the family histories passed down to us; and in our own minds as well. A few of these images are appealing; most are not. Some contain elements of truth; others consist almost entirely of falsehoods. Although these images inaccurately reflect the realities of illness, they acquire a reality of their own as they are imposed on sick people, and an even greater reality when we use them to define the roles we play. Here are some of the images of the sick person that affect the society and culture surrounding the person with CFS.

DRAMA AND ROMANCE

Chronic fatigue syndrome, we read, strikes down its victims in the prime of life. It's the mystery ailment.

To the extent that a chronic fatigue illness has an image of mystery and drama, the image draws on the old image of tuberculosis. Tuberculosis was common in eighteenth and nineteenth century Europe and took on a Romantic cast when artists, writers, or poets were among those who contracted it—the famous example being Keats.

This image of the sick person as languishing poet is a powerful one that died neither with Keats nor with the nineteenth century. My own obsession with tuberculosis testifies to its appeal. If you have to be sick, have what Keats had. Instead of just lying in bed, languish. Never pass out: swoon. Maybe the truth in this image is that since you have to be sick anyway, you are entitled to do with your sickness whatever you can manage to do.

A second disease in the mold of which ours is sometimes cast is cancer. In both cancer and CFS, the cause is complex and mysterious, the treatment far from reliably curative, and the image of the sick person far from the romantic idealization of the languishing poet. Since no one knows why we are ill, it is easy to imagine that the cause lies in ourselves. Besides, if no one knows what made us ill, who knows for sure that we may not contaminate everyone else?

The third disease to which CFS is sometimes compared is AIDS. "The CFIDS problem will not go away. It is real. It seems to be on the increase, and, if so, its relationship to the AIDS epidemic will need to be investigated with great urgency," said Dr. Paul Cheney in a statement to a Senate subcommittee. The same subcommittee heard testimony from a representative of Minann, Inc. (a medical advocacy, research, and information foundation), who quoted a CFS patient in Florida as saying: "My health insurance premiums doubled when the insurance company interpreted CFS as a disease 'similar' to AIDS." (Both of these statements appeared in the Spring 1989 issue of *The CFIDS Chronicle*.)

In reality, how is CFS like AIDS? First, AIDS is caused by a virus. CFS might or might not be. Second, the public images of the two illnesses are, on the whole, negative. If people with AIDS are portrayed as sinful, people with CFS are portrayed as neurotic and lazy. The distorted image of AIDS as the contemporary biblical plague readily pulls in CFS as well. Everyone knows what those people did to get AIDS, the image seems to say. What did you people do? And what's it going to cost the virtuous?

THE SAINTED MARTYR

In the romantic image, illness is poetic. The sick person is creative. In the image of the sainted martyr, illness is a cross bravely borne by a physical weakling of superhuman spiritual goodness. The disease lays waste to the body, but raises the soul, creating a special relationship with God. In the image of the sick person as sainted martyr, this ailing slave of duty carries on despite pain, fever, and all kinds of other symptoms that debilitate the rest of us.

There is no question that spiritual beliefs can help people to find meaning in illness and strength to deal with it. People can also use illness as an opportunity for spiritual development. On the other hand, the fact that I am not religious did not in any way prevent me from playing the role of sainted martyr or, perhaps more accurately, the slave of duty. The vicissitudes of an unexplained illness are such that you sometimes cannot help feeling like Job. On a more mundane level, there are times when you force yourself to do things you are plainly too sick to do because you do not want to let anyone down, because you want to be a good person. If playing the role of martyr is the only way you can keep your promise to take your children to the zoo, or the only way you can finish a report you said you'd finish, or the only way you act the way you think a decent human being should act, then it's not such a bad role.

We do our best, but we aren't martyrs, and I would like to suggest that when we present ourselves to the healthy world, we avoid encouraging the distortion of the illness to this image. Don't we just want to been seen as ourselves?

THE HEROIC WARRIOR

In the heroic image, the targets of the mystery plague are warriors rather than victims. Instead of illuminating your mind or uplifting your soul, an illness apparently does wonders for your guts. The people idealized in this image are sometimes so strong that it is almost impossible to believe that they are sick at all. Whatever they have must be very different from what I had and what you have. Their illnesses are such exciting adventures that you almost want one yourself. The language magazines and television movies use to foster this image of illness includes words like "fight" and "conquer" illness, or "win the battle" against it. The most courageous warriors take on even greater challenges. If you have a disability and you want to be a heroic warrior, you do the gutsy impossible. Run marathons. If you have a disease, vanquish it.

Heroic warriors are so successful in resisting illness that their battles practically never include tactical retreats. They usually win the war, and, if not, they have the satisfaction of fighting the good fight. They are not scared or tired. They are Hercules, only sick. The battles they fight are time-limited and winnable, and during the battles, fighting is their only activity. To be a heroic warrior, you need a large independent income and terrific household help, because going to work every day, getting the laundry done, and driving your children to their piano lessons certainly interfere with waging war.

If you know what you have and that it's here to stay, a lifetime commitment to the role of heroic warrior means trying to defeat an unconquerable illness instead of trying to coexist with the illness so that you can pay attention to more important things. For someone with chronic fatigue syndrome or another strange illness, playing the heroic warrior is a different matter. It is sometimes useful, particularly when the object of the fight is to preserve whatever you can of your former life in case you get well; or when the object is to find out what's making you sick. Heroic or not, keeping your job, taking part in family life, and maintaining interests more interesting than illness are battles; so is making sure that doctors are your active allies in the search for help.

I also think that there's a little truth in the idea that illness toughens you up. I used to be a real baby about fever and pain. If my temperature went above 99.0, I'd curl up in bed until it was 98.6 again. In the midst of my chronic fatigue illness, I had an ovarian cyst rupture. My temperature went up higher than usual and so did my white blood count, but except for noting the pain in my side, I didn't feel much worse than usual and I did everything I ordinarily do. I'm tougher than I used to be.

GOOD PATIENT/BAD PATIENT

Good patients get in bed and pretty much stay there, compliant and uncomplaining, until their health is restored. They rest, drink lots of liquid, and follow their doctors' orders. They remove themselves from daily life, never attempting to participate in the activities of healthy people. They are cheerful. They are grateful for the flowers sent by kind friends and for the effective help offered by their doctors. Bad patients are cranky complainers who refuse to rest, drink insufficient amounts of liquid, and disobey doctors' orders. They get just what demanding, help-rejecting whiners deserve: they remain sick.

The role of "good patient" is difficult for someone with a chronic fatigue illness because playing that role requires the complementary role of "good doctor," a role that includes, among other things, effectiveness. For someone with an undiagnosed illness, the role is almost impossible. Even though an illness may simply not be diagnosable, the doctor who cannot diagnose it thereby becomes a less than perfect doctor. He can't tell you what you have. He can't really help you. The doctor's inevitable imperfection—frustrating to doctor and patient alike—makes it impossible to live up to the role of good patient.

THE MANIPULATIVE MALINGERER

Manipulative malingerers are spoiled brats who use the pretense of illness to live the soft life. Alex's CFS forced him to leave his job. When Alex's company denied his claim for disability benefits, and when Social Security twice did the same, he encountered this image in its most vivid form. Nothing says more clearly: the only thing wrong with you is that you don't want to work.

Of the people I know who have chronic illnesses, not one plays this role, but practically everyone reacts against it. Lest they be thought malingerers, people keep going when they belong in bed.

They don't ask for help when they need it. The minute I started to feel at all well, I was ready to accuse myself of malingering. "If you have it, you're a malingerer," Ginny says angrily. This image of illness is especially harmful to people with CFS because they often appear healthy to others, who easily assume they are just lazy.

THE NEUROTIC

"Oh, I thought that was psychosomatic," a neighbor recently remarked to Ellen. Dr. Stephen Straus, a well-known researcher at the National Institute of Allergy and Infectious Diseases, shares the neighbor's view. In a 1988 article in the *Journal of Infectious Disease*, he writes, "An early hypothesis regarding the etiology of the chronic fatigue syndrome is that manifestations represent somatic expressions of a psychoneurosis. It is impossible to completely dispel the notion that the chronic fatigue syndrome represents a psychoneurotic condition. On the contrary, there are observations that support the hypothesis."

There can be little debate about the negative impact of Straus's views on the public image of chronic fatigue syndrome and the lives of sick people. In the Spring 1989 issue of the *CFIDS Chronicle*, Marc M. Iverson points out the consequences of Straus's published claims: "Patients are viewed as morally deficient, symptoms are not taken seriously, medical and legal claims are hard to defend, employment opportunities are limited, and the focus that should be placed on 'organic' research is displaced." In other words, the negative impact of Straus's claim is so powerful and so pervasive that not only are CFS sufferers sometimes considered neurotic, but research into the physiological causes of the illness is slowed down considerably.

Is chronic fatigue syndrome a neurotic symptom? If researchers psychologize the illness and do not look for organic causes, we'll never know otherwise.

THE NEUROTIC WOMAN

A refinement of the image of the person with CFS as a neurotic is the idea that CFS is a disease of neurotic women. The neurotic woman image meshes perfectly with the image of the Yuppie overachiever as well as with traditional stereotypes of women: stressed by the work world where we don't belong anyway, women combine natural weakness with a propensity for neurosis in this somatic symptom. We should have stayed home. Or would that be malingering?

CFS really is diagnosed much more frequently in women than in men and apparently affects more women than men, as do MS and lupus. Men, however, certainly have chronic fatigue syndrome and other chronic fatigue illnesses. To men, this image offers a double whammy: you have an imaginary ailment of neurotic women.

THE BURDENSOME NON-PERSON

This is the image of the chronic invalid, the sick wife who spends all day everyday in a darkened room, contributing nothing to her marriage or any other relationship, but requiring expensive, tedious care. Since good patients get better and she remains sick, she is a bad patient. In novels—and I'm calling her "she" because in novels, she usually is—her husband has an affair, and since the invalid wife is more a burdensome object than a person, you end up sympathizing with him. It is often unclear whether the invalid wife is really sick or only a malingerer or a neurotic. When the image of the burdensome non-person changes so that the individual acquires a personality, it is usually a nasty one.

The burdensome non-person is usually a wife, but sick husbands and wives are apparently equally afraid of fitting this image. Becoming a burdensome non-person means bringing worse than nothing to the marital relationship; it means that the healthy spouse would be better off with you dead.

When I was sick, my husband made it clear that he preferred having me alive and sick to having me dead, but the truth is that although I did not become a nameless object locked in a sickroom, I was burdensome. It is burdensome to have a spouse whose limited energy limits your life together. I no longer did what I thought was my fair share of the work. I am lucky to have a husband who thought that the unfairness of illness had descended equally on us.

Single? You, too, can see yourself as a burden. "I wanted to know who I could turn to in a time of sheer terror in the middle of the night," Alison says in speaking of her friends. "Because my issue was: I'm too much for you. How am I going to know what you're feeling? How are you going to set limits with me?" Singles are afraid of placing too much of a burden on any one friend and also of losing all their friends if the illness drags on too long.

TYPHOID MARY

For people who are ill and who do not know the causes of their illnesses, the Typhoid Mary image is a threatening, scary one: if you don't know what's making you sick, you don't know for sure whether or not it is contagious. The doctors I saw all seemed convinced that my illness was not contagious. Neither my husband nor my daughter nor anyone else seems to have caught it from me, but I still worry. I wouldn't eat from my own plate if I didn't have to. If my husband or daughter says, "I don't feel too well," my heart pounds and I hover around until it becomes clear that my husband ate too many chili peppers or my daughter has a cold.

I was luckier than I knew. "There's this world of primitive fantasies and fears that I found myself having to put words to," Alison tells me. "I worried that if I had saliva contact, that could be dangerous. One of my friends has two kids, and I'm really close to them. When we'd share meals together, which we did regularly, she wanted to keep separate dishes. And the way she explained it to me wasn't sitting down and saying, 'I'm really scared.' It was more, 'How contagious is it? I don't want you making food.' It built up. I could see it in her face. I gave her a lot of information as soon as I knew what was going on, but there wasn't a lot of talk. It really built up to the point where I felt she had the sense that the viruses were sort of coming out of my body. It came out in feeling, and it was hard to get her to put words to it. I was just furious. I think she couldn't believe she was feeling this way, but she was. A lot of little things would come up, like I'd touch a piece of food, and she'd be afraid that I'd contaminated the food. So we kept separate dishes. I think her biggest fear was that her kids would get sick."

During the pregnancy of one of Ellen's friends, the friend's husband was afraid of contagion. Later, "he was afraid to have me take care of the baby. I stopped kissing people. I stopped sharing food," she says.

Sometimes we worry, and our friends don't. "I didn't think this was contagious until I heard a doctor speak," Kay says. "He was pretty clear that until we know what this is, we can't be sure it won't be transmitted through saliva, kissing, or whatever. I was seeing this guy, and I told him that. He just kissed me, which was the best thing he could do."

ILLNESS AS A CHARACTER DEFECT

One image of illness is caused by the belief that the sick person's mind and body are a unity. If only the sick person would understand that he is making himself sick, this view holds, he could change his lifestyle, adaptation to the world, character structure, or, in short, himself. He would then become well in body and mind.

One of the reasons Andy doesn't talk to people about his illness, he says, "is that I don't want their opinions. I found people's opinions extremely unhelpful. I always feel that there's an attitude about it: how are you creating this? And if you could only find, insightfully, how you're creating this, you could free yourself from it. And I find that totally unhelpful as a way of supporting me in my journey to get better or to deal with not getting better. I had a friend say, 'Until you understand the benefits of the illness that you're creating for yourself, you'll continue to be sick.' It's a terribly hostile thing to say. Even if it were true, it's not going to help me." Andy is a psychotherapist, as are many of his friends, but he discovered a similar attitude in the world of alternative healing. "A psychic said to me, 'Well, you know the underlying reason is a pent-in emotion, and yours is rage.' I don't believe in that one-to-one correspondence between emotion and physical illness. I don't believe things are related in such simplistic ways."

One variation on this image occurs in the idea that people with certain personality types resist illness, while people with other personality types attract illness in general or attract specific diseases.

The absence of a solid, familiar, explanatory diagnosis makes people with chronic fatigue illnesses the perfect blank screens onto whom to project this image of the mental weakling; and the psychology of unexplained illness makes people with no diagnosis especially likely to project this image onto themselves. Someone with a mysterious illness is the perfect victim to blame.

POLLYANNA

One of the role models the character-defective sick person is supposed to emulate is Pollyanna. People simply will insist that believing that you will get better must be a self-fulfilling prophecy, that thinking can make it so.

Before the discovery of streptomycin and isoniazid, optimism was considered the key to success in curing tuberculosis. The newsletters for tuberculosis patients in Saranac were full of injunctions to think happy thoughts. The favorite contemporary targets for this ideology of curative optimism are people with cancer. Since it is difficult for healthy people to believe that those with chronic fatigue syndrome and undiagnosed or vaguely diagnosed illnesses are really sick, it becomes especially easy to enjoin us to believe our illnesses away.

The bare fact is that to believe you are getting better when every objective and subjective sign says that you are not getting better is psychosis, not optimism. To criticize people for not believing something they have no reason to believe—and criticism it is— is cruel: the absence of solid information about what made you sick and whether you will ever get rid of it is incredibly confusing. It is very hard to be realistic about something when you know almost nothing about it. The result is a sharp longing to know what is really going on and to distinguish wishes from facts.

The big cruelty of the think-it-away ideology, however, is the risk of thinking that the illness is getting better or going away. You have good mornings, days, weeks, or even months. What you learn from them is not to set yourself up for disappointment. A good day is cause for hope, but to fool yourself into thinking that one good day means the end of the illness is almost a guarantee that the next bad day will be one of unnecessarily deep depression. "My worst times are times of feeling better and then, for reasons unbeknownst to me, starting to feel bad again," says Kay. "I can't ever put my finger on anything I've done that makes me feel bad again, so it feels totally out of control. It sort of has a life of its own in my body."

It is true that happy, optimistic people, sick or well, feel happier and more optimistic than do sad, pessimistic people. Genuinely optimistic people with baffling illnesses, however, run the risk of being so certain that the illness is going away that they make much less effort to find out what it is than do realists or pessimists. Furthermore, since it is by no means clear that people can become happy and optimistic just by trying, and since illness does not naturally bring out the Pollyanna in most of us, playing Pollyanna often means passing yourself off as the opposite of how you really are. Therein lies the little truth in this image: almost everyone with a chronic fatigue illness fakes health, energy, and good spirits, at some point, often for a good reason.

THE CLEVER MANAGER

The clever manager image, which dominated my own struggle with illness, typically arises in stories about people's relatives. "Oh, my cousin had Epstein-Barr," you'll hear. "She had to learn to plan everything and re-arrange her whole day. She needed to sleep every afternoon from one to four, so she changed her work schedule so she could work in the morning and the evening. . . ." This image is, I believe, the most powerful one of all. It is positive, attractive, and believable. It seems to offer a way to live happily and productively with the illness. It promises control over the illness and, perhaps best of all, a sharp distinction between the illness and the person who is ill.

In this image, the hypercompetent Wonder Person, blessed with the good fortune of a predictable illness, anticipates the ups and downs of the illness and arranges life accordingly. Tired every afternoon at precisely two o'clock? The clever manager schedules his day so that his nap begins at two o'clock. Apparently he has previously arranged to have a job that leaves him free to nap in the afternoon.

His children do not arrive home from school in the mid-afternoon. His freezer is stocked with meals that he pops into the oven on days when he is too sick to cook.

The clever manager makes a list of tasks to be accomplished. He assigns priorities to the tasks. He analyzes his own energy level in relation to time, and he performs each task at the time at which he has the appropriate energy level. He has, naturally enough, cleverly managed to contract an illness that leaves him the mental energy to do all this organizing as well as enough physical energy to perform the top priority tasks. I gather that he does mind giving up frivolous, low-priority pursuits. Or maybe he schedules them in somewhere, too. This paragon accepts his illness and adapts realistically to it. In fact, the clever manager has such complete control over his illness that unless you happen to know he's sick, neither you nor anyone else, including his spouse, children, and employer—he still has one— could tell there was anything wrong with him. The clever manager is never a nuisance to other people.

This image of the clever manager perfectly expresses today's Yuppie values: even if you're sick, you can still have it all. The image also represents healthy people's wish to deny that what has happened to you could happen to them. It lets them cling to the belief that illness need not change people's lives for the worse

The clever manager image is insidious because it seems to promise a desirable role you could potentially play. Encountering the image usually means encountering guilt that you are not coping with your illness as well as other people cope with theirs. In fact, the role is one sick people already play, although often not very well because it's hard enough to be sick without having to be perfect, too. If only we could really get organized, we could contain our illnesses and minimize their impact on our lives. If illness had no impact on our ability to get organized, we'd probably all be clever managers. I would have been. I tried all the time.

RESISTING THE IMAGES

These images of the sick person provided by our cultural, family, and personal histories are not at all what we would like to use as mirrors for the new selves we become in chronic illness. Nonetheless, these images are the only ones we have. Part of our adaptive struggle is coming to terms with the lack of fit between images of the sick person and the images we have of ourselves. In our innocent efforts to adapt to illness, we often find ourselves playing roles defined by images we do not like; and we increase the burden of illness by using attractive features of the images to create unrealistically high standards of how we should adapt.

You may not be able to change the images of illness that pervade the culture around you and that will surely affect other people's reactions to your own illness. But you can try. And, at a minimum, you can recognize them as what they are, just images, and avoid mistaking them for what they are not, reality.

4

It's Just Fatigue:

MYTHS ABOUT CFS

In the course of my illness and then my interviews with people who have CFS, I have come across a number of myths about the illness. Healthy people, as you might expect, have some misconceptions about CFS. But people who have the disease often seem to believe myths of their own.

SOCIETY'S MYTHS

The myths I describe in this chapter are often healthy people's defenses against the unwelcome realization that what has happened to the ill can happen to the healthy. The problem with these myths, however, and the reason I devote space to them here, is that they make chronic fatigue illness worse than it need be. Recognizing these myths for what they are—defense mechanisms, and just plain misconceptions about the disease—may offer, I hope, something akin to the relief of finding a name for the illness.

Feeling Tired? You Must Have CFS

One of the worst myths concerning chronic fatigue illness seems to be rooted in something I call "illness amnesia," the inability of healthy people to remember what it is like to be sick. People are able to remember that they were sick. People also remember particular symptoms, including pain and fatigue. What they generally seem to blot out is the most central sensation, namely, the sense of malaise or illness itself. The appearance of that feeling lets you know you're coming down with something, and its disappearance lets you know that you're recovering. The vivid memory of the universal sensation of feeling sick is precisely what vanishes in illness amnesia. This leads to one of the central myths about CFS: that it is a sense of fatigue rather than a real feeling of having a real illness.

Feeling tired and feeling sick are quite distinct sensations. Nonetheless, Roseanne tells me, people say to her, "I'm getting what you have. I'm tired." Ginny's father told her: "Gee, I've had this all my life and I never knew it!"

Chronic Illness Teaches You a Lot

It really does. You learn a lot about having a chronic illness. I also learned to drive and cry at the same time. Others, including Wendy, feel that illness has forced them to examine what they really want from life. The point is that although some people use illness well, illness itself doesn't necessarily teach anything important. This myth can be harmful because it puts pressure on you to learn important life lessons at a time when it seems all you can do is just to get the laundry done.

The Worst Times Are the Only Times

People who knew that my temperature reached its peak in the afternoon would sometimes say, "Oh, so you work in the morning when you don't feel sick." Actually, I did feel sick in the morning. And at night. This myth is a good example of illness amnesia. Human body temperature happens to peak in the late afternoon or evening. Almost everyone has had the experience with a mild, ordinary illness of feeling better in the morning than in the late afternoon. Having an illness seems almost always to mean feeling a little worse, then a little better, then a little worse, then a little better, but there is a big difference between feeling a little better and feeling well. Healthy people forget that having an illness often, although not always, means feeling rotten morning, noon, and night, all day and everyday.

In the first year of her illness, Leah tells me, "I'd been so burned by people experiencing me as inconsistent and unavailable and unreliable." "The ups and downs were difficult for people, understandably," says Ellen. What's an up? There's variation among people as well as variation within any one person's illness. For Roseanne, "when I get my own breakfast and lunch, that's a good day." Nonetheless, when Roseanne's closest friend was planning her wedding, she insisted that Roseanne, who is partially bedridden, be her maid of honor. "She suddenly denied the illness. She ordered the dress! I know it's her problem. She can't deal with it, and she wants to make me well for that day," Roseanne says.

CFS Should Stay on Schedule

One of the feats of cleverness that clever managers pull off is to contract predictable illnesses. In so doing, they make life hard for the rest of us because people expect us to know how sick we will be at specific times in the future. "Will you be able to . . . ?" and "Will you feel like . . . ?" and "Will you have the energy to . . . ?" always used to upset me. In truth, I usually had very little idea of how sick I would feel. Committing myself to some uncertain prediction of my future energy meant committing myself to do whatever I had said I would do even if my prediction was wrong.

Any ability to predict how sick you will feel almost makes matters worse for healthy people because it confuses and misleads them. It is probably more fair to others—and more honest—to explain and even insist that you just can't predict how you will feel at any given point in the future.

You Should Be Able to Control CFS

Since getting little sleep, eating badly, and maximizing stress will make most people feel crummy, taking good care of yourself should certainly allow you some control over how sick you feel. To some extent, it does, but it worked only one way for me. Staying up very late almost certainly made me feel terrible, but getting plenty of sleep was no guarantee at all that I would feel comparatively well. All it guaranteed was that I wouldn't feel quite so terrible as I would have if I had stayed up late. That's all. It is very discouraging to eat a good dinner, relax, sleep from eight o'clock in the evening until seven o'clock in the morning, and then feel really sick. It is discouraging and unfair, but it happens. The truth is, no matter how you try, you can't totally control the symptoms of CFS; that unpredictability is part of the frustration of living with the disease.

If You're Here in Public, You Must Be Okay

Attending this party was your choice. You're here, and you're talking to people, so you must be okay, or so healthy people assume. Actually, chronic illness can be almost indescribably boring. And the feeling of being left out is even worse than the feeling of boredom. Sick people's presence at parties and other social occasions often means that overcoming lonesomeness has taken priority over overcoming illness—alone. It does not necessarily mean they are well.

Attending a party is at least a choice. Going to work usually is not. Nonetheless, people assume, if you're going to work, you must be okay. "Especially for the first year," says Leah, "I was working all the time, so a lot of people didn't understand that that was all I was doing. For the better part of three years, I went to work, and I came home, and I went to bed. Even though I told people that I was sick, I don't think there were many people who really understood what was actually happening."

If You Aren't Complaining, You Aren't Sick

"People think: He was sick," according to Andy. "The idea is that he did get sick, and now that he doesn't talk about it anymore, he's probably better."

Alison tells me that her mother recently said, "Oh, I thought your headaches had gone away."

"Real denial," says Alison. "And I think there was a time when I probably set everyone up for that because I was using denial just to keep my job. The idea of something being chronic is the hardest thing for people to understand, especially when I look all right. What I get is: 'You look really good!'"

Chronic Illness Makes You Rich

Although I have never heard anyone say outright that chronic illness makes you rich, many people must assume that it does because they say: "Why don't you take some time off?" "Maybe you need a long vacation." "Have you tried staying home for a while and taking it easy?" "Why don't you get someone to come in and help you with that?" People say these things out of genuine concern, but hearing them always made me wonder whether there wasn't some wonderful philanthropic foundation somewhere that sends its agents all over the country to look for sick people. One lucky day in the near future, one of these agents would ring my doorbell and walk in, followed by teams of gardeners, maids, and nannies. Also accompanying the agent would be an accountant who would not only straighten out my taxes and bills but would pay them as well. The truth is that people with CFS might want to take time off or hire help; they just might not be able to afford it.

You Now Have Plenty of Free Time

"One of my closest friends wanted me to pick her up at the airport," Kay says. "I think her idea was that I wasn't really doing anything, so why not? She said, 'I don't think you're pushing yourself enough.' And then I realized that she and other people probably didn't have the foggiest notion of how I was feeling. It wasn't that I absolutely couldn't pick myself up and drive to the airport, but it would be like doing that with a 103 degree fever and the worst flu you ever had. You could do it, but it would be a tremendous strain." As Alison says: "People think you're not working, but illness is a lot of work. There's very little time when you feel good."

Everyone Gets Better

This one breaks my heart. Healthy people have, by definition, never stayed sick. Their concept of illness seems to include only two outcomes: you either die or you recover. To have a chronic illness is to be reminded that besides heaven and hell, there is also purgatory.

The myth takes two forms: first, the belief that you will recover and, second, the optimistic conviction that you are now recovering. "Oh, but you'll get over it!" "You'll be well by next summer!" "But you're not as sick now as you were last winter!"

When an illness is undiagnosed or called something like chronic fatigue syndrome, the situation is complicated because the expectation of recovery is questionable. Some people with chronic, presumably viral illnesses get worse. Some get better. Some stay the same. As author Cheri Register points out in *Living with Chronic Illness*, an insistence on recovery certainly can be depressing if it is a reminder that you may never recover. It may make you wonder whether you have something so horrible that a brave front of cheery denial is all that's expected of you. It may also act as an assurance that the painful uncertainty of the illness has been completely misunderstood.

Everything Is the Same

According to this myth, everything about the sick person and his or her life is just the same as before, except, of course, for the minor matter of the illness. This myth usually emerges in comments and questions revealing the assumption of healthy energy and competence. That assumption really hurts because it is a vivid reminder of loss. "Your garden must be looking great after all this rain." "How's your work going?" "With your skills, you won't have any trouble finding another job." For Kay, who loves her job, the loss of the ability to work was painful. "I had a friend who said, 'So when are you going to get on with your life?'" Kay tells me. "I wasn't working. I said, 'I am!' As if there was something else I could have done!"

Encountering this myth is also painful because it sharply reveals the extent to which people see you as the same person you were before the illness. In reality, of course, the loss of that identity is the biggest loss of all. "This is the one that really got to me," says Leah. "I've always been generous with my time and energy, and retrospectively I realized that I was sort of paying for maybe having done too much of that in the past. It seemed to me that there were a number of people who were asking me to be my whole, generous, pre-illness person, people who didn't get it that everything I did cost something."

Sick People Do Not Want Sympathy

If sympathy lets you know someone else cares that you are sick, there's nothing wrong with it. Furthermore, the mental dangers of a chronic fatigue illness include blaming yourself for being sick and feeling guilty because you are not fulfilling your responsibilities. A friend's expression of empathy, sympathy, or compassion can be very powerful because it can arouse feelings that counter the self-blame and guilt. Someone else's compassion can awaken a compassion for yourself that has nothing to do with self-pity but acts as a reminder to be less demanding and more gentle to yourself. Although a get-well-quick card is the wrong choice, a conventional expression of good wishes during illness may be a validating gesture to someone whose illness is often minimized or denied.

All CFS Patients Want Any Suggestions They Can Get

Actually, there are two myths about sick people's wish for suggestions: all suggestions are welcome, and none are. Some sick people clearly do not like to have suggestions spill in. Other people, however, welcome at least some suggestions, and some take the happy attitude that they can use all the potential help they can get.

Some healthy people are energetic clippers and senders of articles. I wish now that I had kept a count of the number of articles I have received on chronic Epstein-Barr virus. People also tell you all about television specials on strange illnesses and stranger remedies, and you hear all about friends and relatives who had illnesses similar to yours. They even urge you to try cures that did wonders for people with problems totally unlike your own. On the other hand, some people are so afraid of causing offense that they either offer no suggestions or apologize for tactfully proffering perfectly reasonable ones. How welcome or unwelcome suggestions really are depends, first, on how the recipient feels about receiving suggestions. It also depends on how they are offered. My dear friend Meredith once showed up at my house bearing a lasagna, her precious old teddy bear, and a bottle of a health food remedy called "Cyclone Cider." The lasagna was practical help. The teddy was a sign that she cared. The Cyclone Cider was a joke, since Meredith knew how tired I was of being urged to try acupuncture, aural readings, and herbal remedies. People care about you! Lighten up! That's what she meant. It was a welcome suggestion.

OUR OWN MYTHS

So healthy people harbor deep untruths about illness, but the illness puts you in touch with reality, huh? People with CFS are exposed and vulnerable to healthy people's myths about illness, but we also seem to have a few of our own.

The Idealization of Ordinary Health

According to this myth, the absence of illness guarantees a constant superabundance of energy and good spirits. Health is not just the ordinary state of not feeling sick; it is great physical strength, emotional stamina, mental energy, clear spiritual vision, and the efficient organization of daily life.

One subsidiary myth is the glorification of just how energetic, emotionally stable, organized, skilled, and altogether terrific we ourselves used to be. Before we were sick, we did everything we were supposed to do and never forgot anything. We were thoughtful friends, model employees, dutiful children to our parents, perfect parents to our children, and loving, considerate, hard-working spouses. The second subsidiary myth is, of course, that if we ever recover, we will once again become such paragons. Just as healthy people suffer from illness amnesia, sick people suffer from health amnesia. Recovery cures it.

Everything Is a Symptom

A corollary of the myth that health means radiant, robust, uninterrupted well-being is the belief that any deviation from physical, mental, and emotional perfection is yet another symptom of the illness. In fact, not every headache is a symptom of chronic illness; people in ordinary health get them, too. Anxiety, crankiness, moodiness, and other emotional reactions, too, are sometimes just that, emotional.

Yes, chronic fatigue syndrome has a bewildering array of symptoms, and the objectively verifiable symptoms are mild enough so that we are readily accused of imagining ourselves ill. If we insist on adding to the list of symptoms every discomfort symptomatic of the human condition, we are not going to increase our credibility.

You Can Diagnose Yourself

Many of us "have" several diseases in our search for a diagnosis. I had subacute bacterial endocarditis until two echocardiograms and numerous negative blood cultures convinced me to abandon it. I then had trichinosis. That was a remarkable self-diagnostic coup because you get trichinosis from eating meat and I had not eaten any meat for nine years. I recovered from trichinosis after a negative blood test.

Tuberculosis was my most persistent self-diagnosis. I sometimes had myself almost convinced that I had it. How convinced? When I had been sick for only a month or so, I had a tuberculin test and a chest x-ray, both of which failed to reveal tuberculosis. About five months later, another tuberculin test missed it again. Only a few months later, I was sure that a third test would be positive but too embarrassed to plead with my doctor for one. After a number of phone calls, I managed to locate a public clinic at a local hospital, where I had a third tuberculin test, which was again negative. I no longer "have" tuberculosis: I was eventually given a special kind of TB test with second strength tuberculin, and that negative result convinced even me.

What made tuberculosis a useful self-diagnosis is that skin tests really can be misleading, so this is not the kind of self-diagnosis that a doctor can readily steal from you. My mild obsession with tuberculosis also persisted partly because it was truly not an impossible diagnosis. Chronic tuberculosis in places outside the lungs really can keep people sick for years and can fail to show up in tests. But, of course, not very often. It's a difficult diagnosis for reality to disconfirm, so if you are desperate for a diagnosis, it's not a bad choice.

Not everyone with a chronic fatigue illness fixes on tuberculosis, but most people adopt a series of illnesses and rehearse Lyme disease, parasitic infections, hyperthyroidism, and many others. Amazingly enough, some people eventually turn out to be right.

You Will Never Recover

Some chronic fatigue illnesses are, in fact, eventually diagnosed as something other than chronic fatigue syndrome. Some are cured. Some go away. Nonetheless, as Norma says, "You feel like you may never get better."

The strong resonance of the permanence myth is evident in the questionnaires mailed with applications for membership in CFS or CFIDS support organizations. Having defined myself as recovered, I find it impossible to fill out questionnaires that ask: how long have you had CFS? What symptoms do you have? I need room to write that I'm not sure what I had, and to write just what Ellen says: "I don't think of myself as sick. I have lingering symptoms."

The belief that the illness is absolutely permanent, can, of course, signal deep depression, and most healthy people interpret this belief as a sign of hopelessness. Believing in recovery, however, has its down side also, since the prospect of recovering can seem so wonderful that even thinking about it makes the present worse than it already is. On the other hand, subscribing to the belief that the illness is here to stay may, paradoxically, be liberating: it may let you focus on how to get through today instead of wasting time daydreaming about something that may never happen. It may thus offer a little protection against false hope.

According to one version of the belief in the disease's permanence, chronic fatigue syndrome involves a continuous susceptibility to recurrence. Leah describes her illness as "in remission." For myself, I'm pretty much OK as long as I'm careful. Oddly enough, I do say that I *had* CFS, sort of, but I'm also careful. According to my idea of recovery, I had something, and I'm careful lest I get it again or get something else. According to Leah's idea, she still has it, but she has to be careful lest its remission end. Is CFS's permanence a myth? Is our behavior merely superstitious? Neither of us knows for certain, and, believe me, neither of us is going to push hard enough to find a definite answer.

You Are the Target of Attacks

When you are sick, depressed, and broke, it is easy to hear the greeting "How are you?" as a mean thing to say, tantamount to "I don't care about you at all, and I've forgotten that you're sick" or "Pay attention to how sick you feel and how rotten your life is." Similarly, after nine doctors have told you that you don't look sick, a perfunctory "You look great" from a friend can feel like the tenth denial of your illness. If your friends are having a party, you feel that by deciding to have it begin at eight o'clock at night, they are withholding from you the possibility of attending. You feel that medical help is being withheld: you have been sick for four months, but there has not yet been a major international medical conference held to diagnose and cure you.

Many of the myths of the withholding world have some validity. In fact, little research funding is allocated to chronic fatigue syndrome, and some of the available research money is wasted, from the

LIVING WITH CHRONIC FATIGUE

viewpoint of those with the illness, on blame-ridden psychologizing. And healthy people often are inconsiderate. We and our illness, how-ever, are seldom deliberate targets. The myth that we are targets is, alas, the myth that we are more important than we really are.

LIVING WITH THE MYTHS

Just as with the images of illness in our culture, these myths—our own or those believed by healthy people—will shape responses to our disease. We can't change everyone else's beliefs. But we can try to bring our own expectations about CFS in line with reality. And we can interact with those in the healthy world a little more easily once we understand the erroneous assumptions they are making about chronic illnesses in general and about CFS in particular.

But if these are the myths concerning CFS, what are the realities? In the next chapter, we'll take a look at some of them.

5

I Used To Have A Life:

PRIVATE REALITIES

Now that we've looked at some of the myths about CFS and other mysterious, chronic illnesses, what about the realities? While the myths are believed by healthy people as well as by those with an illness, the realities of having CFS are something many healthy people can't readily imagine. But people who have or who have had a chronic illness will instantly recognize these problems—some large, others minor—that come with having CFS.

FEELING PERSONAL DIMINISHMENT

Laura, expresses the sense of a diminished self experienced by so many CFS patients. She and I are drinking tea in the sun-room of her house. She is a dainty, pretty blond woman in her thirties whose eyes sparkle with health. In fact, she has been healthy for three years. For the preceding four years, she says, "I felt ill all the time, queasy, exhausted." She had no energy. "My sense of myself changed," she says. "I felt defective."

Real illness, as opposed to that false image of illness as triumph, forces upon us redefinitions of ourselves that almost invariably connote diminishment. No matter how we redefine ourselves, the redefinitions mean that we are less than we were. If, for instance, we define ourselves in terms of activities or accomplishments, we are less than we were because we really do less than we did. Illness simply does not increase competence. If you are no longer the employee, parent, gardener, skier, writer, cook, or lover you were, you feel you are a diminished person.

Acutely ill, Greg found himself in a work situation that would have been difficult even if he had felt well. "I tried to struggle along," he says. "Had I been well, I probably would have tried to find a job elsewhere. At the time, I didn't have a lot of confidence in myself. I really think this illness erodes your confidence something fierce. You end up in a cycle of being self-defeated because you want to do more. On the days you feel like you *can* do more, you go out and do more. Then you feel sick again. So, eventually, your world's getting smaller and smaller, and you're doing less and less. You never know how you're going to feel when you wake up in the morning."

Faced with these regrettable and maudlin sentiments about personal diminishment, the optimistic healthy person may be unable to refrain from pointing out that personal worth is something entirely separate from everything I've described: personal worth is not a function of how good a provider, partner, spouse, or parent you are. In the eyes of God and good people, a person is just as worthwhile after he becomes sick as he was before. I agree, but that's not the point. What is diminished is not so much a sense of personal worth as various valued parts of yourself, selves you once were, and the diminishment is not imaginary. Furthermore, it is not an essentially depressed, unrealistic lowering of self-esteem. The diminishment is real, and what is diminished is you and your world, not just your good feelings about yourself. "My world has shrunk," Roseanne says.

DISTORTED PERCEPTIONS

A major symptom of chronic illness is a distortion in the perception of effort: everything seems to demand effort, and, in particular, activities that used to seem effortless become demanding. When everything seems to demand effort, it becomes difficult to differentiate between tasks that really require a lot of time and energy and those that do not. Oddly enough, too, tiny differences in required effort become important. The energy required to make a tuna fish sandwich or to make scrambled eggs may seem about the same, but, as I tell Roseanne, there were times when I ate a sandwich instead of eggs because I couldn't summon the energy to wash a skillet. "I can't be bothered even to make a sandwich," Roseanne says. Besides, even if you correctly estimate the effort required to do something, who knows what unexpected and overwhelming demand might crop up? Mailing a letter might not seem like much effort, but suppose your car gets a flat tire on the way to the post office? If you know that you have only the energy necessary to drive to the post office and back, and if you also know that you cannot face having to deal with a flat tire, the task of mailing the letter may seem so overwhelming that you stay home. Small tasks you didn't think twice about when you were healthy suddenly become complicated maneuvers.

LACK OF MENTAL ENERGY

Maya, who turned out to have Lyme disease, describes a vivid memory of a task that demanded more mental energy than she had. The task was buying a birthday card for a friend. The memory is of sitting on the floor of the card shop too overwhelmed by the array of cards to pick one out.

Well, a healthy person may ask, what about priorities? Why not just list the things you have to do and assign each task a priority? Maybe the card has such a low priority that it does not merit a special trip to the shop. Maybe so, but illness gave me a new appreciation of the concept of mental energy. The healthy person, who does not think that trivial tasks like scrambling eggs and mailing letters take any energy worth mentioning, also does not notice that it requires energy to decide which tasks are trivial and which are important. Going to the card shop may seem less demanding than deciding whether or not buying the card is a high or a low priority task.

"Mental energy!" says Roseanne. "I might not even be able to make the list for my husband to do the food shopping. I have to give all my energy to what I'm doing."

DISTORTION OF JUDGMENT

Illness plays havoc with mental organization and judgment. What goes to pieces is not only the capacity to make decisions, set priorities, and organize yourself and your life but also the capacity to realize that your judgment itself has gone to pieces. When I had been sick for about two months, I began writing a paper I wanted to send to an academic journal. I was very interested in the paper and so sick that everything I wanted to say seemed equally important. My judgment was so shot that I had no idea that the paper was as bad as it was. Luckily for me, the editors of the journal to which I sent it spared me the embarrassment of having it appear in print.

One emotional consequence of having judgment go to pieces is vulnerability to anxiety and guilt about things that are plainly not worth worrying about. Small obligations can loom large. You may awaken in the night berating yourself for having forgotten to pay a bill that isn't due yet. Another consequence is what must seem like inappropriate responses to events. After Alison was hit by a speeding bicycle, she found herself in an ambulance. "I thought on the way to the hospital: Oh! I'll get a chance to rest!"

DISTORTION OF TIME

Illness itself, especially fever, stretches time. The low energy of illness makes time drag. Impaired judgment and difficulty in recognizing the impairment also contribute to the distortion of time. To the distortion of time inherent in the illness the medical systems adds the need to tolerate almost unbearable and sometimes frightening delay. In the spring of 1987, for example, there were places where it was necessary to wait a month for the results of an AIDS test. Adaptation to the long, long waiting involved in medical tests worsens the distortion of time in a way that feels especially cruel.

Adaptation to living in a world of stretched time also has its hazards because most of the rest of the world lacks that adaptation. You tell yourself that since this task is overwhelmingly large and will take almost forever, you will sensibly do a little bit at a time. And you do. You do very little. And a tiny bit more. And then a tiny bit more. You congratulate yourself on adapting to your illness. Sure, you haven't finished the task yet, but you are getting there. At that point, someone with a normal sense of time notices that you've hardly begun the task and tells you so. So much for adaptation.

"When I first got sick," Roseanne says, "I'd think: maybe next month I'll be better. Now I think: maybe in the summer."

IMPAIRED MEMORY

People who write about CEBV, CFS, or CFIDS often list impaired memory as one of the cognitive symptoms of the disorder. One possibility is that impaired memory is a primary neurological symptom of the illness. Another is that impaired memory is a secondary symptom, a function of exhaustion. At any rate, forgetting things is a reality of many chronic illnesses. You forget deadlines, birthdays, promises. You forget the important and the trivial. In your effort to compensate for your bad memory, you try to remember to write everything down, but then you forget that. You leave yourself notes that you forget to read. You run out of milk, go to the store to buy milk, and return home, having forgotten the shopping list on which you had written a single item, milk, and discover that what you forgot to buy was milk. You can hardly believe what you've done, and then comes the worst part: if you forgot that, what else have you forgotten? In a state of panic, you check to see whether you really mailed the quarterly payment to the Internal Revenue Service and whether your in-laws are really visiting in two weeks and not tomorrow. Ludicrous as it seems, you worry about what you may not remember that you might have forgotten.

"At one point," says Ginny, "I thought I must have Alzheimer's. I'd lived in this house six years, and I'd forget where the light switches were. I forgot to pick up the kids at school. One morning, we got in the car to go to church, all five of us. I had my coat on, and I realized I had no idea what I was wearing under it! Driving, I'd have no idea where I was. Who did I visit?"

"Now," says Norma, "my ability to read, concentrate, and think is fine. My recent memory may not be a hundred percent. Last summer I tested it out. I had a continuing education exam to take. You read an article and then answer questions about it. I used to have quite a good memory, but at one point, taking the test, answering the questions, I realized it was as though I'd never read the article. So, I realized my memory was still not right. Now, I don't know."

One consequence of a rotten memory is a strong, realistic mistrust of yourself. You learn to suspect yourself of having forgotten things. Another consequence is horribly inconsiderate behavior to other people. You no longer do what you said you'd do because you've forgotten what you said. Furthermore, you sometimes forget so rapidly and completely that no one could be expected to believe that you've really forgotten. You hardly believe it yourself. You are going to a birthday party for a child. On the morning of the party, your spouse says, "Remember? You said you'd buy Rachel's present today." For once, you remember having said that. At six o'clock in the evening, when the toy stores have closed, you again remember. Instead of buying Rachel a present she'd like, you buy whatever you can find at whatever nearby store is still open. That's hard to take when you consider yourself someone who used to be thoughtful.

DIMINISHED SELF-CARE

Some people respond to illness by adding something like a new command to their internal computer programs for living: IF OPTIONAL, THEN DELETE. Haircuts, dental appointments, ironed shirts may all be declared optional and then deleted. Fun is optional. Especially vulnerable to deletion under this command are meals prepared only for yourself. People skip meals or absolutely minimize the effort of food preparation. You eat a sandwich from a napkin or you stand over the sink so that you won't have to wash a plate.

"I had friends who helped me with food shopping and things like that," Kay says. "They volunteered, and I sometimes let them, and sometimes I forced myself to go food shopping. And it would take every ounce of strength I had. I didn't do anything you could call cooking. I defrosted. I put a piece of cheese between two pieces of bread for lunch. I had cereal for breakfast. Anything that took no energy. I lost a lot of weight because I wasn't eating very much."

Leah's illness had the opposite effect: "I wasn't doing anything. I didn't walk more than a block. I was totally physically inactive. And I didn't want to dirty any dishes, so I lived on ice cream." She grins. "Out of the carton. I didn't think about it at all. I wasn't interested in my body. I noticed I was gaining a lot, but I thought to myself, first things first. The first thing was to get myself better. I put on thirty pounds."

Some people succeed in fighting the pull toward diminished self-care by instituting a rigid program of self-maintenance. From the outside, that kind of program may seem like a series of compulsive rituals or like a series of exercises in unabashed narcissism. The person goes to bed at exactly eight o'clock every night and makes no exceptions, even for you. He eats a macrobiotic diet. His hair always looks as if it's just been cut. He knows what he does not do; he knows what he does and when he does it; and he really does it. He fights the same pull toward diminished self-care that we all fight, but he succeeds better than most of us. If such a program works for you, there is nothing wrong with it; I just wasn't able to make it work for me.

DIMINISHED CARE FOR OTHERS

Diminished self-care easily extends to diminished care for others, and, once again, often appears in the form of an empty refrigerator. Food shopping, something I used to take for granted, actually consumes a lot of energy. Worse, planning what to buy and cook requires mental energy. One solution is to shop infrequently and on those occasions to buy huge amounts of canned, dried, or frozen food that requires almost no preparation. I have a clear memory of standing in a supermarket check-out line, looking at my shopping cart, and realizing that the groceries looked like someone else's: instant mashed potatoes, frozen dinners, frozen vegetables in plastic bags, almost nothing fresh or real. To feed yourself on junk is sad, but to watch yourself buying nothing but junk for your growing child gives you a horrible, shameful feeling.

SMALL LOSSES AND LOWERED STANDARDS

"I forced myself to do things, or I just couldn't do things," says Don. "It was hard to say no. Finally, I was forced to give things up and to say no because of relapsing or getting sicker, and I was giving up more and more. It was only when I gave up enough to get sufficient rest that I started to improve."

I used to take great pride in my little yard. Deploring modern low-maintenance gardening, I pursued gardening at its most labor intensive. Instead of tucking in a few marigolds to create a spot of color, I would double dig the soil, add my own compost, and plant delphiniums I had raised from seed. My return was some pretty flowers, lots of exercise, and a sense of personal accomplishment.

Anyone who believes that pride goes before a fall will be pleased to know that mine did. I couldn't even keep the lawn in decent condition, and my flower beds were weedy. I had to lower my standards. Who cared? I did. When I had been sick for three months, the seed catalogs arrived. Realizing that unless things changed rapidly for the better, I would be unable to garden in my usual energetic fashion, I actually cried over the catalogs. I hated the small losses of giving up my beautiful garden. I hated giving up the hours of browsing through the catalogs, making plans, anticipating. I hated every blade of crab grass. The worst part, however, was a new and unwelcome recognition about my cherished garden. Once I could no longer make plans to put in a new flower bed here, to move a shrub there, to add a thick layer of compost somewhere else, I was forced to see the garden only as it really was, not as I eventually wanted it to be. It is just an ordinary suburban yard, and I have lost the harmless illusion that it is special.

CLINGING TO INTERESTS

The loss of interests is a hallmark of depression, and the sick person's deletion of optional activities, especially hobbies and interests, must look from the outside like depression. A chronic illness does not actually mean a loss of interest at all, but grief at the inability to pursue interests and sadness at the resulting lowered standards. "I can only look at the lawn for so long," says Alex, whose wife helped him maintain his standards and his energy: she bought him a self-propelled lawn mower.

It is hard to see yourself becoming someone who used to have interests. The interests remain so strong that you develop sad little efforts to retain some tiny portion of what was once a major pursuit. I had no energy to do my usual yard work, to raise perennial flowers from seed, or to go bird watching; but, I decided, feeding birds really requires almost no time or energy. I have to give up most of my hobbies and pleasures, but I'll still feed the birds. I did, but, there was something sad about it because it seemed to represent what I had left: not much.

Before his illness, Alex was an avid backpacker, climber, and fisherman, but, he says, "that began to kill me." He adds: "It's the loss of a lifestyle. My brother doesn't understand it at all: 'Get you out in the boat and get a couple of beers in you, and you'll be fine!'" His friends, too, want him to join them for canoeing and fishing trips. What's left of that part of his life? He still does some fishing nearby. "But," he says, "it puts me in bed for two or three days."

Muscle pain and stiffness forced Norma to stop playing the piano. "Once in a while," she says, "I test it out. I played yesterday, and I'm OK today!"

OBSESSIVE PREOCCUPATION WITH ILLNESS

You give up many interests, but you may acquire a new one, illness, which can become a demi-god in your life. It looms over everything you do. You read about it, think about it. It becomes a morbid preoccupation. You observe your symptoms; you chart their course; and you look for new ones.

Erik, who shares my single-minded determination to find a diagnosis, outdoes me when it comes to amassing knowledge and sifting it for answers. "I practically had to learn medicine," he says. With some enthusiasm in my voice, I ask him about *The Merck Manual*, but my enthusiasm reveals the superficiality of my medical studies. Erik finds the manual incomplete. He reads journals and textbooks.

When the origin of an illness is unknown, the possibilities offer room for obsession, including the possibility that some offending organism or allergen, the original or a new one, may be lurking around. Ellen and I went through phases of scrubbing our kitchens in chlorine bleach. Marna still doesn't trust her humidifier. Erik thinks he may pay for tests of the air quality in his work place.

TERROR

Between the onset of the illness and the diagnosis of a chronic nonfatal illness, medical poking and prodding nearly always reveal something terrifying. One test shows that there is something in your breast, liver, or lung; but that test does not show what it is. You wait for a second test. You wait for the results. Those are hours, days, or weeks of acute terror. Tired as you are, you can't go to sleep or you awaken in the middle of the night. Eventually you discover that the something is a harmless cyst. The next doctor tells you that he suspects a brain tumor.

Then there's chronic fear: is this thing permanent? Is it getting worse? How long will I be able to keep my job? What is this neglect doing to my children? Is my spouse going to stay with someone so awful? You see visions of the piles of bills you haven't even bothered to open, and you wonder whether the electric bill contains a notice that the power is going to be shut off tomorrow. You see a doctor who tells you to reduce the stress in your life. A new test shows another mysterious something somewhere, and the chronic fear again becomes acute terror. My doctor was once having a hard time listening to my heart because it was pounding so hard. She said, "I don't know whether you're more afraid that I'll find something or that I won't." I didn't know either.

SELF-DOUBT

"I tend to wonder: is it anything?" Marna tells me. Having been told repeatedly that you look fine, that your lab tests are normal, and that the symptoms you report reflect stress, hypochondriasis, or malingering, you may begin to wonder whether you have, in fact, made yourself sick or imagined the entire illness. "Yes, I have my doubts sometimes," says Andy. "I wonder if there is something going on with me that's creating this, but my deepest belief is that I am not doing this to myself, emotionally."

Thalia has felt comparable doubt about her daughter Marcie's illness, which various doctors and school officials have sometimes labelled school phobia. Thalia has considered that possibility. "For the sake of my child, I didn't want to overlook anything," she says. Although a psychiatrist who examined Marcie said that the problem was not psychological, and although a doctor had diagnosed Marcie as having CEBV, Thalia took her to a psychologist, who tested Marcie and concluded that she was definitely not school phobic. Even so, until a friend of Thalia's came down with CFS and described the illness as Marcie had done, some doubt remained: was Marcie really sick?

GRUMPINESS TOWARD THE HEALTHY WORLD

As your illness becomes a demi-god, almost a new person in your life, a nasty second self, "a cloud over the house," as Roseanne says, it becomes difficult to remember that it is a force largely invisible to most other people. Amazingly enough, it hardly enters their lives.

That discrepancy between how important the illness is to you and how unimportant it is to most other people seems to generate some feelings almost as nasty as the illness itself, for example, a petty vulnerability to small hurts. Healthy people acting in perfectly reasonable ways can generate petty resentment. Leah says: "There was a change in me, so I spent a lot of time being angry and petty and feeling grumpy and feeling bad because I'd been so generous in the past."

Why aren't those people helping me? Can't they see how sick I am? It would be so easy for them to do this, and it's so hard for me! Why can't people be quiet so I can rest? Thoughts like these are a common result of having a chronic and debilitating disease.

LIVING WITH CHRONIC FATIGUE

A SENSE OF HELPLESSNESS

Perhaps the most depressing experience of a chronic fatigue illness is the sense that nothing you do makes any big difference. You sleep for twelve hours and awaken feeling worse than when you went to bed. Or you sleep for twelve hours and feel infinitesimally better than if you had slept for five. You take aspirin, and your fever goes up. Or your fever goes down, but you feel sick anyway. Your urgent, desperate need for help in knowing what the illness is has no influence whatsoever on your doctors. Even if you really know that there is some correspondence between what you do and how you feel—many people eventually do identify a correspondence—there are times when the correspondence seems worthlessly small.

"As a younger person," says Andy, "I had a strong belief in my ability to control the world, including thinking I could beat diseases. If I had a cold, I would just resist it! I didn't get sick much, and I took pride in that. I've realized that I'm not in control of my body, and I'm not my body. My body's going to rot, and I'm something else."

DEATH WISHES

At the worst times, I felt that there was little left of me except illness. I looked with a sweet longing at on-coming buses. Fortunately, I always remembered that a person was driving the bus, a person who did not need the responsibility of having run me over. I would start to enumerate the reasons to live. The first was that I would never, ever leave my daughter, and I would certainly not leave her to live with a mother's suicide. That's as far as I got: suicide was not an option, but the wish remained.

I think, however, that although what I sensed was a strong wish to die, the wish was really an impulse to kill the illness, not to kill myself. Somewhere in my fantasies of dying was always an image of myself awakening, recovered from illness. I think that the wish also represented a rejection of the self the illness has forced upon me, a lazy, cranky, dependent, stupid self. Regardless of what the wish represented, it was there, and one of the many rotten things about it was the pressure to keep it to myself. To have to live with a sick person is bad enough; it would be completely unfair to increase the burden by talking about wanting to die. So I kept it to myself most of the time, but sometimes I selfishly let it out. My husband, reading a newspaper article about AIDS, remarked, "You know the only good thing about AIDS?" I can't remember what he actually had in mind, but to my shame I remember that I immediately replied, "Yes. You get to die."

For Leah, too, the thoughts of death are tied to a loss of self, in her case, the independent self who works: "I thought that if I stopped working, I would kill myself." She begins to cry as she talks to me. "The essential image I have of myself is of someone who can take care of herself, economically. Not rely on anybody else. Without self-sufficiency, I don't care if I have life. It is my life. I gave a lot of thought to what would happen if life was always going to be like this. I had a time limit. I was quite serious about it."

BECOMING OVER-EMOTIONAL

Chronic illness can generate an emotionality that looks like hysteria. Any long illness is, of course, good cause for tears, and some doctors are easily able to incite any rational person to frenzied madness, but the emotionality of illness feels like some raw, primitive force, not like a response with a reasonable cause.

There were times when I decided to get out of bed only because I could not stop crying. Anger erupted easily. I was sharp, cranky, and nasty. I snapped at my daughter for doing things that it would be abnormal for a teenager not to do. It is normal for teenagers to listen to music with lines like "There's something about you, girl, that makes me sweat." A teenager who arrives home from school at four o'clock to announce that she has left a crucial homework assignment and book in her locker and needs a ride back to school is acting perfectly normal. In any case, the appropriate maternal response is to maintain a calm so zen-like as to make the Buddha appear hyperkinetic and not to yell, "Turn off that horrible music, and don't ask me to do anything!" Then I would be pathetically sorry and ashamed. Especially when I'd been cranky with my husband, I became overwhelmed with gratitude for his forebearance; the last thing a psychotherapist needs to come home to is one more emotionally volatile person. Then I'd go to bed, not because I was sicker than usual, but because I was unfit for normal life; I put myself in isolation to protect other people from my horrible behavior.

Because angry outbursts and, indeed, any strong emotions are exhausting, some people conserve their limited energy by minimizing any emotion that might be tiring. "I made a decision that I was not going to experience any emotional upset," says Leah, "and, on the whole, I kept it. So, all my relationships shifted. I stopped fighting. I didn't have an argument for twelve or fourteen months. The consequences were terrible because when I cut out the disagreeable part, I cut off the other end of the range at the same time. My emotional range became extraordinarily constricted."

Leah's was a decision. Others find that they simply lack the energy to argue, disagree, or confront people. Greg bore up with a difficult work situation in part because he was "not able to cope and confront things that were going on. The energy wasn't there." I found myself becoming more agreeable than ever before in the literal sense that I expressed agreement. Whenever possible, I told my husband that I shared his opinions, liked his suggestions, thought he was right. He must have thought I was losing my mind.

DISAPPOINTMENT IN PEOPLE

One of the most valuable illusions of health is the belief that, if times were ever really tough, everyone would come through for you. Your friends and loved ones care so deeply for you that they would be wonderful. They would really help. No one would let you down.

The reality is that people cannot quit their jobs and desert their families to do your cooking and shopping. Kind people cook one or two meals, but that's usually it. They do not take your cat to the vet. They do not take out your trash. They do not pay your bills. Even when they do their best, it's hard to realize that what you can expect from other people is very little.

Some people do come through. "People are wonderful!" says Kay, whose friends shopped for her and otherwise gave her consistent support.

But some friends really let you down and, in doing so, destroy precious illusions. In an early phase of Ginny's illness, her church helped with meals. "This is what they do," she tells me. "One winter, for four weeks, I didn't have to cook a meal. It was a help beyond words." The next winter, the church members again helped for six and a half weeks. "And, to have that visitor, that contact with the outside world!"

Eventually, however, church members expected Ginny to recover and resume her contributions to the church's activities, yet she could not. "We had to leave the church, and we lost most of our close friends," she says with deep sadness. "We couldn't fulfill our quota for attendance or continue to be active. We were politely ostracized. We'd given so much! And I'd forced myself to be there so many times! It seemed like blackmail: either you do this, or you're out. I go to another church now, and I see the faces there, and I ask: will they do that to us, too? No one in our new church knows about my illness. And to explain to the kids why we can't go back to our old church! It's like losing a family. It was the most devastating thing for my husband, too."

DISTRACTIBILITY

I have at last reached one of the few positive realities of illness: It is possible to be distracted from illness, and distraction helps. Although I am reluctant to make connections between illness and character, I think that one of the few benefits of a baffling illness may be to make people good listeners. If you are sick and tired and your life is going badly, it is just wonderful to hear about anyone other than yourself. Other people go to interesting places and have interesting stories to tell. You learn that an effective way to fend off an unwelcome "How are you?" is instantly to ask, "How are you? What have you been doing?" With any luck, you then have the pleasure of hearing about someone else's life instead of your own.

Frivolous as it may sound, my illness is also responsible for introducing me to a wonderful distraction, namely, the Boston Celtics. Before I was sick, I just hated spectator sports. I liked to do active things, and I had no interest in sitting in front of a television watching other people play some stupid game. Once I was sick, I was too tired to do anything very active. Just to spend some time with my husband, I started collapsing in front of the television while he watched what I now recognize as the greatest of all basketball teams, our Celtics. I started watching. I loved it! It was impossible to attend simultaneously to my illness and Larry Bird.

On a less frivolous note, Andy says: "There is a certain gift of the illness in that you cannot get so hung up about your career and your this and your that. You pay more attention to treating yourself well. The quality of your life is more important. The quality of your health is not."

APPRECIATION FOR OTHERS' CONCERN

Before I was sick, I would never have believed how much other people's caring would matter to me. If I heard that someone was sick or was having some other kind of trouble, the first thing that came to my mind was a fear of intruding: "Oh, she wouldn't want to hear from *me*" or "I might do something wrong, so I'd better do nothing." I cannot describe how glad I am that many of my friends know better than that. Along with a sometimes terrible emotional vulnerability came an openness to help, an ability to let myself feel helped by the knowledge that other people cared. People did not have to do anything except express concern.

UNCERTAINTY ABOUT YOUR OWN LIMITS

To have a chronic fatigue illness is to live in a state of normlessness or lawlessness. There are no rules. There aren't even any absolute guidelines about what's good for you. The rule I would have liked is one that would have told me when to keep going and when to quit. On a visit to the Boston Museum of Science, my daughter bought a little plastic card that is supposed to measure your level of stress. You hold your thumb on a spot on the card for sixty seconds. If the little spot turns black, you're under extreme stress. If it turns blue, you're relaxed. There are a few colors in between. I wanted a card like that, a gauge, but instead of telling me how stressed I was, it would have told me when to rest and when to struggle on. If the little spot turned black, I would have known to go to bed. If it turned blue, I would have known to keep going even if I felt rotten. As it was, I kept going when I could because I was tired either way.

"People say, 'Why don't you rest?' I'm depressed if I'm home in bed," Marna reports. "I'm ambivalent about looking for work now, but it's not so depressing. I need a lot of structure." Norma, too, has kept going as much as possible. "Maybe I would have recovered faster if I'd stayed in bed," she says, but she felt that the people she worked with were her "second family."

Although I began to recover after I stopped working, I am reluctant to admit that the obvious connection exists, and I never quit pushing myself. I worked in my garden, did housework, shopped for food, went to parties, and otherwise expended every bit of energy I had. According to many people, I should have stayed sick. "Push it and you get worse," says Erik. Don agrees. But to me, resting when I could possibly have been doing anything was quitting. It was accepting the illness. I was convinced that if I gave up and went to bed, I might never get up again.

I was lucky. I had a choice. Kay, Meg, Roseanne, and many others much more acutely ill than I ever was have spent weeks in bed because they were too ill to do anything else. Furthermore, my all-or-none thinking about the conflict between fighting the illness and giving in was misguided. Kay and Greg's time off from work did not lock them into a lifelong pattern of chronic invalidism. Both took time off, rested, and recovered enough to return to work. They differentiate between physical rest and psychological submission in a way that I did not. In announcing that she has a chronic illness, Leah takes a tough stance that proclaims her intention to fight for herself. Similarly, Kay succeeds in making her illness a "backdrop," not the center of her life, yet she says vehemently of her illness: "I *don't* accept it. I want it to go away."

ILLNESS AND EGO

A psychologist might condense these private realities of personal diminishment, cognitive disorganization, poor memory, emotional hypersensitivity, and the like into the statement that a chronic fatigue illness poses a threat to ego function. Ego, in that sense, means something more than self-esteem, and it means something we all need, namely, the capacity to organize inner experience and outer reality so that we have a positive, continuous sense of who we are in the world. A baffling illness means not only a change in the perception of who you are, but many genuine, negative changes in yourself. It is a narcissistic injury: it injures not only good feeling about yourself but also the bases of that good feeling.

A mysterious illness is especially threatening to basic ego functions because one such function is "reality testing," in other words, differentiating between outer reality and inner fantasy. A baffling illness, by definition, impedes reality testing. Since no one knows what the reality is, there is nothing solid against which to check fantasy. If your left thumb starts to hurt, you have no way of knowing whether you're imagining the pain, whether it is a sign of something other than your baffling illness, or whether it is a diagnostic clue. The chances are good that no one else knows either. It is hard to maintain a sense of a continuous self when you are unpleasantly different from the way you were and when neither you nor anyone else knows what to expect.

The point of this rather depressing discussion is not simply to add ego weakness to the list of symptoms of chronic fatigue syndrome. Rather, the point is, I hope, a potentially helpful one, namely, that most of what is offered to people in the name of help is, in reality, unintentionally aimed at weakening our already threatened ego function. Consider the advice that we accept our illnesses. Accept what? Personal diminishment? Impaired judgment? A sense of time that makes a day feel like a week? People with chronic fatigue illnesses do not really need a lot of help acknowledging the seriousness of the problem. We do need help in cultivating selective denial. We need distraction. Most of all, we need help in reality testing, especially help in understanding what the illness is and what to expect from it. We need good research. We also need support from each other and from our friends, families, and the rest of our social networks. The need for support is so great that illness can become a new, unwelcome member of our social worlds, an unwelcome membership that is the topic of the next chapter.

6

Losses And Gains:

FAMILIES, FRIENDSHIP, AND WORK

The particular social realities and dilemmas of a chronic fatigue illness vary greatly from person to person. This great variation is not surprising: the specific issues we face depend upon the varying social worlds we inhabit. In his twenties, Erik is trying to plan his career and make a decision about marriage even though he has no name for his illness and no ability to predict its course. As single people living alone, neither Erik nor Don nor Alison faces Ginny and Ellen's dilemma of trying to care for young children during an energy-deleting illness. The family support given to Marna by her husband and children is unavailable to people living alone, who, however, escape the strain that illness imposes on a marriage. But marriage, friendship, and professional life are all affected when you have a chronic illness. Since you are never sick in a vacuum your primary relationships will all be influenced by your experience. Knowing what to expect from your spouse and family, your friends, and your boss and co-workers should make it easier to cope with the social realities of CFS.

FAMILIES: STRAIN AND SUPPORT

Alex says that during one of the worst phases of his illness, his wife would run out of the house to get away from him.

"It's a huge strain on the family," says Ellen. "More than you could imagine."

"The dynamics within a family!" says Roseanne. "There's strain on the marriage and the family. My husband and daughter are supportive, but their lives have changed. Everything revolves around my illness. If you didn't have a strong relationship to begin with, you'd wind up in divorce."

A spouse or partner, then, is something of a mixed blessing during illness. On the one hand, the presence of a partner guarantees, at the very least, that the ill person does not spend the days, weeks, or months of an acute episode in total isolation from other human beings. At best, a partner is that one other person in the world who totally believes that you are ill, and a family is the support you need. "My husband knew I wasn't making this up," says Norma. "He could feel I was sick." In explaining to me her reasons for not staying with a support group, Marna says of her family "I *have* support!"

Partners, however, like parents, children, and close friends, may need to protect themselves against the recognition that the illness is as bad as it is. "My husband denied some of my illness," says Ellen. Since illness falls on couples and families, it is fantasy to imagine that partners are immune to the entire range of nasty responses experienced by the ill person. If we have trouble differentiating between ourselves and our illness, if we feel anger, frustration, depression, self-doubt, and all the rest, how could our partners be exempt? Furthermore, healthy partners are not necessarily exempt from the distorted images and myths of the general public. Like everyone else, they may take personally the unpredictable vicissitudes of the illness, expect predictions about the immediate and distant future, and greet memory lapses with incredulity.

The Lack of Privacy

For the ill person, one difficulty posed by living with a partner or family is the lack of privacy in which to fall apart. The presence of a spouse and children may constitute an implicit demand to pull your-self together, shape up, and act at least a little bit healthy and cheer-ful. The demand may at times feel overwhelming. Awakening cranky and exhausted, with my eyelids swollen and my temperature up, I sometimes wanted the privacy to not be seen like that. I wanted not to have to say how I was that day. On the other hand, there were, of course, times when the mere knowledge that I was not alone in the house offered some feeling of comfort. On weekends, I'd hear my daughter talking with her friends. My husband would be watching a football game on TV. Life was at least going on.

Shifting Roles

The role of lover? Not this year, dear. I have a headache, fever, and swollen glands. I can't stay awake, but I don't sleep well, either. Leah comments, "Sex? Forget it."

Still, we struggle to remain who we were, to maintain our roles in marriages and families, to continue to do our share. "My normal day runs fourteen hours," Ginny says. "When my husband's here, he helps out a lot, but he travels. I handle all the finances, and we'd get behind and have late charges. My husband would offer to do the laundry, but what he could do with a washing machine was a miracle."

After Alex became too ill to keep his job, his wife continued to go out to work. She also helped Alex to organize his time and energy. Every week, he makes a list of things to accomplish, and he takes pleasure in completing the work. Eager not to burden his wife, Alex has accepted her suggestion that he take responsibility for some household tasks. "Do you mind doing the laundry?" she asked. Although aware that this new role is not a macho one, he didn't mind. "The washing machine said: large capacity." Alex laughs. "So I packed it in, and it walked across the kitchen. I put new jeans in with a white shirt. I hope tie dye comes back because we have a whole wardrobe."

Difficulty Parenting

The urge to be the responsible, capable, nurturing parent you were may be especially strong. Dissatisfied with their children's experiences in the local public schools, Ginny and her husband had reluctantly moved their children to private school. "And we're paying a fortune in taxes," she says. Besides, even though she participates in a car pool, she still has to drive 300 miles a week to get the children to and from school. Once she was ill, there were days when she was simply not well enough to drive at all, and the children lost time from school. Furthermore, when she did drive, she was terrified that, in her weak and disoriented state, she would have an accident.

In trying to continue to put the children's education ahead of her need for rest, was she nonetheless risking their safety? If she had moved the children back to the local public schools, would she have been sacrificing their education to her needs? I don't know whether she asked herself those questions. In her place, I would have. I also wonder about the ease with which such a conflict could become a marital one. What happens when one spouse's illness requires a change in the lives of the children?

Perhaps the strongest testimony to the strength of the wish to parent despite illness is people's willingness to go ahead and have children. Ellen, who became pregnant while she was ill, found that her pregnancy seemed to improve her health. In the second trimester of her pregnancy, she stopped running fevers. Furthermore, she says, "my attitude became more positive. I had hope." By the end, she felt so well that she thought that the illness had gone, and although she was exhausted after giving birth, for the year since that time she has had only isolated symptoms of the illness.

How does anyone with chronic fatigue syndrome take care of young children? Ginny gave me one answer: "My mother has basically raised our youngest child. She's wonderful, but I felt he was becoming more hers than mine." Recovered, she adds: "But we're all set now."

And how is it possible to explain the illness to young children?

"Do your children have some understanding of what's been going on?" I ask Greg, whose young children have greeted me as I arrive at his house.

"I don't think so. Three years ago, I was home for half a year. They could see that I was here, that I wasn't going to work, and they adapted. We tried to make them understand that I wasn't well, that I couldn't do some things I wanted to. When I was home sick, I spent most of the six months flat on the couch. I'd get up, barely get through breakfast, and I'd go to sleep on the couch until lunch time. I'd be able to rouse myself for a little lunch, then I'd pass out on the couch. Then everybody would be home. It was very difficult."

Laura, now fully recovered, was raising her young daughter while she was ill. Her daughter had always been the kind of child who could happily spend time alone in her room. When Laura, a widow, was ill, it was easier to allow her daughter to follow that pattern than to urge her to take up sports or other activities that would have required Laura's active involvement. She now worries about the long-term consequences of encouraging that pattern of staying quietly at home.

It is easy to imagine that children in or close to their teens, with the mental capacity to understand an illness and the physical ability to offer practical help with chores and such, might offer greater support and fewer demands than young children. Yet with the ability to understand come worry and fear. The older child or teenager, then, continues to need attention but may also need reassurance that the illness is not something worse than it really is. Norma says of her daughter, a young teenager during the acute phase of Norma's illness: "She didn't relate to it as a real thing. She knew I was tired all the time. She'd try to cheer me up. But a good part of her denied it. I spent more time with her. At first, I needed to be left alone, but after a while, I began to see that my family had to be my priority."

It can be difficult indeed to remember that the denial is a defense, especially when it alternates with bubbly, wonderfully effective efforts to cheer you up.

MORE MIXED BLESSINGS

The knowledge that an ill person lives alone may, it seems, trigger caretaking in friends and in the community.

"People gave me things," says Alison, "people who could see through the illness to the person."

"I live by myself, so I spent lots of time just by myself." Kay is describing an early, acute phase of her illness. "I wasn't bored because I was too sick to be bored, so I really spent my days just lying in bed, reading when I could, and watching TV. And my friends were all wonderful." When she was hospitalized, friends in distant parts of the country flew in to visit.

Laura, a single parent with a young child, found strong support from her church, whose members came in to feed, bathe, and care for her child, especially when Laura's daughter developed mononucleosis while Laura herself was still very ill.

In contrast, the knowledge of a partner's presence may lead people to believe that such caretaking efforts are superfluous; the partner, no matter how burdened, creates the illusion that you already have someone to take care of you. Leah describes that situation: "No one ever brought a meal the entire time. I was sort of shocked."

Friends may understand neither your illness, nor the extent to which your partner suffers from its impact, nor the strain it puts on the relationship. To the shame and guilt you already feel about being sick, you add shame and guilt about inflicting the illness and your ill self on your partner, who may feel ashamed and guilty about not bearing up cheerfully, not welcoming the chance suddenly to become the sole support in what used to be a double income family, and not joyfully doing all of the household chores you used to do.

SINGLE PEOPLE AND NEW RELATIONSHIPS

Erik has been asked repeatedly whether it really matters what he has because none of the likely possibilities is curable anyway. "When I try to nail down details, I'm told it doesn't matter." It matters to him because he needs to know what he can expect. "I'm twenty-eight," he says. "My decisions about career and marriage depend on my health."

"I've certainly questioned relationships with men," Kay tells me. "It's hard enough to meet men and get into a relationship, and to have this added on makes me feel kind of flawed. It's different with friends I've known for a long time. But if you're talking about a long-term relationship with someone, who's going to buy into living forever with someone who has a flaw? That's an issue in my life. I've gone ahead and had relationships with men, but nothing serious. It's still a big question, how much I let it affect me. I wonder how lovable I am."

Laura was still ill when a relationship with a man did become serious. Before then, she had been able to adapt her life to the illness and limit its perceptibility to other people by harboring her energy. "I felt ashamed of being sick," she says, and she developed a lifestyle that enabled her to hide the illness from most people. She never stayed up late, never scheduled more than one activity on any weekend, always put her daughter to bed at eight o'clock, and then nearly always went immediately to sleep herself. When she entered a serious relationship with a man, however, she began to see herself and her pattern of living through his eyes and began to realize the extent to which the illness was limiting her. Furthermore, as she became close to him, she was unable to disguise the illness, and he was ambivalent about having a relationship with someone who has so little energy for anything. Laura's story, I might add, has something of a storybook ending: she recovered from her illness and married the man.

SOCIAL LIFE

"I *cannot* go out to a restaurant." Roseanne speaks emphatically, as if she's had to press the point before. "It's exhausting. So many people have asked me to go out to lunch, and they've taken it personally when I can't go. I've put friends on hold. Some of the mothers of my daughter's friends have reached out, but I haven't wanted them to know me the way I am now." Roseanne's illness started suddenly, and she senses a sharp discontinuity between the person she was and the one she is now.

Greg, in contrast, believes that he has had the illness off and on during most of his life. When I ask him about his social life, he says: "I've never had what one would call an active social life. In college, I did very little. I always used to think of myself as not particularly outgoing, but I'm not so certain any more. Even now, I rarely can cope with being around crowds of people, the smoke and everything."

Many people, however, neither put friends on hold nor experience the relative continuity Greg describes. Rather, people try, in one way or another, to maintain that part of their lives. A major impediment to doing so is the need to confront the various images and myths of the illness as they manifest themselves in personal encounters. People will ask how you are. They will tell you that you look great. In so doing, they will raise the dilemmas of whether to talk about the illness or whether to reveal it at all.

TALKING ABOUT THE ILLNESS

"I absolutely avoid talking about it," says Ginny. "At first, I tried, but no one wanted to hear. In this society, when people ask 'How are you?' you are supposed to say 'Fine.' Even sympathetic people don't understand. They get tired, too. It's like childbirth: there are books, but you can't explain it."

"I used to talk about it more," says Andy, who now never talks about his illness and, in fact, encourages the belief that he is well. "I don't remember the decision, but, in retrospect, there must have been a decision just not to do it any more. I don't know if that came with the idea that this may be my way of life. I realized that I was talking about my illness a lot, and I felt: this isn't happy. The more I talked to people, the more I was focusing on it." Meg sounds like Andy: "I don't like talking about illness. It's not a fun topic."

In contrast, when Leah describes the decision to manage her illness, she emphasizes the importance of announcing to people that she has a chronic illness: "I felt that I wanted to be seen accurately. Going public about the illness helped me to deal with that discrepancy between how I was seen and how I experienced myself." Having informed people about the illness, however, she too prefers to let it recede to the background: "With people who acted as if it was business as usual, I had to keep talking about the damn illness because it was like a negotiation. Something had to happen first for regular life to go on." Raising Ginny's theme of the impossibility of expecting real understanding, she adds, "Maybe for them, it hasn't happened yet."

For Kay, as for Leah, the point of talking about the illness is to reach a point where she won't have to talk about it any more: "I don't have frivolous friendships. I have good friendships. I never felt

LIVING WITH CHRONIC FATIGUE

that I wanted to hide stuff from my friends. You don't want to burden any one of them, accepting favors. They know this is a part of my life, and we talk about it and then get beyond it. It's a prerequisite to everything else."

FRIENDS IN NEED

"Key parts of my friendship network just dropped right out of my life." Leah is in tears as she tells me about it. "Nina backed way off. Annie kept insisting that nothing was happening. She just stopped returning my phone calls and insisted that there was nothing wrong. I'm actually so angry about it now, past anger. And I had a number of opposite experiences of people I never would have asked for help just coming in and doing wonderful things, sending notes and letters."

I had some wonderful experiences, too. Neighbors with whom I am friendly but who are not close friends presented me with a beautifully arranged basket containing a card, books, and gourmet delicacies that required no cooking. This is from a letter sent by a couple I knew only slightly: "For almost a year now we have been keeping abreast of general news about your health from several mutual friends who have shared our concern. We kept our interest off to the side so as not to intrude. We would like to let you know directly, now, just how much our thoughts have been with you during this trying time." I cried.

HOW IS YOUR WORK GOING?

In listening to people tell me about their struggles to keep working despite worsening illness, I have again and again realized that the image of the malingerer is precisely the opposite of the truth. To keep their jobs, people drop virtually every other part of their lives except sleep until living is reduced to working, sleeping, working, sleeping. Forced to stop working, they long to return and judge their progress by their readiness to do so. Unable to work, they wrestle with guilt and the loss of self-esteem, and they return to work when they are far from well.

Susan Conant

For Andy, Leah, and others who are self-employed or who otherwise lack access to any kind of disability benefits, one reason to keep struggling is obviously financial necessity, but it is not the only reason. Leah says outright that her career is her life. Even in the worst phases of her illness, she managed to work two and a half days a week. Marna, for whom work is not an absolute financial necessity, first cut down her hours, then took a full-time job. That job ended, and she is now job hunting. Work means, if not actual health, normal life, functioning in the world, contributing, participating, doing your part, maintaining an identity.

Showing Up

"It was difficult," says Greg, "because I was in a difficult job situation. My company has a very strong health department, but I didn't go to them early on. I was dragging myself in come hell or high water. I tried to struggle along. I would not give in to it. I felt it was important to show up and fill a space. I continued to get sicker. I reached the point where it was taking all my energy just to get myself to work, all my energy to get home, and I was not doing anything in between. Fortunately, my job situation was such that nobody really caught on."

Issues of Competence

The accusation of malingering is especially unjust because the decision to stop working seems to be based not on the perception of illness but on the perception of the inability to do a job. In general, I did not hear people say that they were too tired, sick, and miserable to keep their jobs; I heard them say that they couldn't do the work any more. Roseanne first tried to return to work full-time, then tried cutting back. "Even part-time, eleven to two, I couldn't concentrate," she says. "I loved my job, but it became impossible. People didn't really understand. I didn't know what they thought. That I could have tried harder?"

In a similar way, people who keep working throughout the illness worry about the quality of their work. "It was so hard to think, concentrate," says Norma, a nurse practitioner. "I was new, so they didn't know I was capable of better work."

The need to keep working despite a sharp recognition of the decreased quality of the work may mean that the illness leaves an unpleasant legacy. About a year after her illness began, Laura was "functioning again, but in a minimal way." Functioning badly or well, she had to complete the final work on her latest book. "I did the minimum," she says. "I feel embarrassed about that book. It's like a first draft, virtually unedited."

As Roseanne, Greg, Norma, and Laura all suggest, one of the disconcerting accompaniments to the unmistakable perception that the quality of your work has degenerated badly may be the recognition that no one else seems to notice the change. Roseanne's boss wanted her to stay. Laura's publisher issued the book that now embarrasses her. If these people don't notice how bad our work is now, we may ask, did they fail to notice how good it used to be?

Ellen's employer, in contrast, noted the change in her work and noted her absences. "I noticed I was tending to make mistakes at work," she says. "I wasn't feeling well. I had cognitive problems, trouble understanding instructions. I was reversing figures." Several months later, still sick and exhausted, she developed pleurisy. She took a week off from work to recover, but she did not. The company for which she worked was a small one. "I was fired," she says. "He laid me off so I could get unemployment. He had to. He needed someone to do my work."

Up to a Point

Employers who are supportive, even compassionate, about short-term sick leave may change their attitudes when employees fail to meet expectations of prompt recovery. When Meg was originally scheduled for the surgery that marked the beginning of her illness, she told her employers that she would be away for about two weeks. She now feels that she should have warned them that her absence might be longer: "It was my fault, too. They were pretty understanding up to a point." Her surgery took place in March. By the end of

June, she was warned that if she did not return to work soon, she would still have a job of some kind, but might well find that it was at a much lower level than her usual one.

Even when a company's official position is outstandingly supportive, individuals within the company may be less so. "Other people's experience of the company has not been quite as good as mine," says Greg. "I was very aggressive in managing my issues. I know a person who was on short-term disability and was being harassed by phone calls from his manager saying, 'Get back here! I know you're not sick!' If he had just told the health department that he was getting these calls, they would have stopped. It's considered harassment. My manager, who also did not believe that I was sick, was told that he could not have any contact with me. He told me point blank that he did not believe that I was sick. He was trying to fire me."

As Kay shows, even a well-intentioned individual in a supportive company may find a long absence difficult to tolerate. "My boss at the time," says Kay in speaking of her six-month absence, "who's still a good friend of mine, was very good, although she was ambivalent because she's a workaholic, and she wanted the work to be done. I couldn't give her a day when I'd be back to work, so that made it very difficult for her to plan. We tried for a while having me bring work home, but it didn't work. After a while, she started to lose some patience, and she said, 'Well, I can't hold your job forever.' I told her: 'You need to do what you need to do. I can't tell you when I'm going to be better,' as much as I wanted my old job back."

ALL OR NOTHING

Leah, Marna, Norma, and others have found it possible to keep working because they have been able to adjust their hours, sometimes decreasing or increasing the number of hours they work. One of the ironies of publicly funded disability systems is that they are all or nothing systems. Either you are able to work full time, or you are totally disabled, and if, in filling out application forms, you even suggest that you can sit upright for ten minutes or lift a twenty-pound weight, never mind declare that you could work part time, you are almost certainly going to be declared ineligible.

RETURNING TO WORK

The myth that going to work means that you are just fine may permeate our own thinking in such a way that we do not anticipate the ups and downs of returning. Greg's return to work was simultaneously a return to a difficult situation he had lacked the energy to manage before his leave. Although Kay returned to a much less difficult situation and to a job she loves, the return was still far from easy: "I had one false attempt. I thought I was ready to go back. I remember waking up in the morning, washing my hair and being exhausted. And lying down, and getting up, and putting on my clothes, and lying down, and finally driving to work and being so exhausted and being afraid that I couldn't walk from my office to the cafeteria. I wanted so much to be back at work. And when I was home, I wasn't really doing anything. I was resting. I didn't have a good measure of how much energy I had, and I clearly didn't have enough for that. That was awful. Another month passed, and I tried again, and by that time, I really did have enough energy to barely get myself there, spend a few hours, get myself home, and just lie exhausted for the rest of the day. Slowly I just worked back into full time."

JOB HUNTING: SHOULD YOU DISCLOSE YOUR ILLNESS?

The dilemma of when to disclose a disability is an important one for people with major disabilities who are looking for work. If a lawyer is applying for a job, should her resume say that she can't see? If you use a wheelchair, do you risk making an appointment for a job interview only to discover that the building where you're to be interviewed is inaccessible to people in wheelchairs? There are no easy answers to those questions, and people often have definite, strictly personal opinions about how they want to handle the situation. It is a particularly complicated issue for people with a chronic illness because passing for healthy is relatively easy to accomplish, at least initially, if the disability is not readily perceptible. The issue is further complicated by the almost complete absence of information about what you're covering up when you disguise the illness. If you don't know for sure how healthy or ill you are, what can you tell a potential employer?

Before Greg took short-term disability leave, his work situation was so difficult that, had he been healthy, he would have looked for another job. When he returned to work, the situation was as he had left it, and his manager, forbidden by the company to contact him during his leave, assigned him low-level work and otherwise made the return far from easy. Greg, however, handled the situation assertively and, with the encouragement of the personnel department, sought a new job within the same company. As I listen to him, I wonder about the impact of his illness on his prospects for a different job, and I ask him about it. He was lucky. People did know about his absence but attributed it to surgery he had had that was unrelated to the illness. He was thus able to skirt the issue of disclosure.

Marna is job hunting now. "Do you tell people about the illness, in job interviews?" I ask. "No!" she says, horrified. "No! No!"

Norma found support for not disclosing her illness when the long commute to her job became more than she could manage and the prospect of a job close to home suddenly arose. "The medical director where I worked gave me a pep talk," she says. "He said the illness had no effect on my work and not to mention it, so I decided not to mention it."

DISCLOSING: PUBLIC ISSUES

Mia favors full disclosure: "If people know I'm sick and they can't deal with it, that's their problem."

Erik, however, points out to me that in some circumstances, maintaining confidentiality about the illness may be an important form of self-protection. He tells me of a woman with chronic fatigue syndrome who found herself unable to get life insurance because of some reference to "brain lesions" in a description of the syndrome. Furthermore, he tells me, some medical insurance plans require that the patient applying for reimbursement for medications sign an agreement to release medical information. Erik advises that it is possible to strike out the release agreement, initial the change, and receive the reimbursement; or to agree to release only the information about the particular prescription. He also warns that the medical insurance plans provided by some employers notify the employer whenever the insurance company pays for a claim. Erik suggests, then, that tests to rule out some diagnoses, including AIDS, might best be paid for by the patient and done anonymously.

LONG-TERM IMPACT

Unlike Roseanne, Alison, Kay, Alex, and others who experience illness in sharp contrast to preceding health and energy, Greg says that he has had the same illness off and on for most of his life. Now, in his late thirties, he reflects on the impact his illness has had on his work life and social life: "There are certain kinds of work that I've avoided because I know that I physically can't take it. The energy level is not there. I couldn't be on the road as a salesman day in and day out. I don't recover quickly enough. And certainly the lifestyle of sales people—eating out, alcohol—I just can't do it. Long ago, I found my way to things I knew I could do even when I was sick, and I limited myself to those. It's part of the disease process. I'd like to do more, and I'm starting to find things I've missed in life, starting to find things I could have done that I missed because I didn't feel well."

Some whose illnesses suddenly interrupted career ambitions and apparently fixed life courses, however, do not regret the change necessitated by the illness. "I was on a career path I'm not so sure I want to be on now," says Leah.

I am surprised. She has made it clear that to call her career-minded would be a gross understatement.

"Now," she continues, "I feel as though I can do it, but I'm not so sure I want to."

So strongly did I resent being told to think of my illness as a challenging opportunity to live differently that I hesitate to admit that illness offered me a new career. I hate to admit it, but I can't resist a happy ending.

Susan Conant

Like a lot of mystery readers, I'd always thought what fun it would be to try to write a mystery some time. As you can imagine, illness offered me a lot of hours in which I was fit to do nothing more taxing than read mysteries, so I read even more of them than usual. After I had begun to recover, I had time to find out whether it really would be fun to write a mystery. Since I was attending dog training classes every week, I decided to set the mystery in the world of dog training and dog shows. Well, writing a mystery turned out to be even more fun than I'd thought, and for the first time in my life, I could babble on about dogs as much as I liked. The publisher who accepted my first mystery must like dogs, too, because I was offered a contract not only for that first book but for a series of three others as well. Damn those smarmy people. They were right.

7

Vitamin C and Bee Pollen:

THE SEARCH FOR A REMEDY THROUGH ALTERNATIVE TREATMENTS

Because CFS has no known cure, people with the disease often spend months or even years searching for something that will at least improve if not entirely alleviate their conditions. For many people with a chronic illness, this search includes forays into the world of non-traditional medicine. How much of homeopathy, acupuncture, vitamin therapy, or neutralizing to try is an individual decision. I didn't experiment too much with this kind of thing, for reasons I will go into later on. But a lot of people with CFS do, and their experiences, good and bad, can give you some insight into what to expect and what to beware of should you decide to look into non-traditional approaches to curing the illness.

HOMEOPATHY

One familiar non-traditional system is homeopathy. This system of medicine was founded in the late eighteenth century by a German doctor named Samuel Hahnemann. It remained popular throughout the nineteenth century, when it offered a gentle alternative to the practices of the "age of heroic medicine," for example, blood-letting and the administrations of heroic (i.e., large) doses of purgatives, emetics, and drugs like calomel (mercurous chloride, which produced mercury poisoning).

Contemporary practitioners of homeopathy argue that homeopathic medicines, called "remedies," continue to offer a safe alternative to the harsh practices of conventional medicine ("allopathy"). In homeopathy, the right remedy for a symptom is the substance that produces the same symptom in healthy people. If you have a sore throat, the right remedy is thus a substance that makes a healthy person's throat sore, but the homeopathic remedy contains only a minute amount of the substance. In this gentle approach, less is more.

So-called homeopathic remedies are available in health food stores, and there are numerous untrained people who claim to prac-tice homeopathy. Since it takes a real homeopathic physician at least an hour to interview a patient and begin to work out the right match between the patient and the remedy, it seems unlikely that reading the labels on over-the-counter remedies will achieve that match. Furthermore, it seems to me that an untrained person practicing any kind of medicine is still an untrained person practicing medicine. In contrast, a trained, licensed homeopathic doctor is a physician as well as a homeopath. If you decide to try homeopathy, be sure to find a trained and licensed homeopathic doctor.

THE SEARCH ITSELF CAN
BE THERAPEUTIC

When I walk into Andy's office, he is just finishing a phone conver-sation. He says good-bye and hangs up.

"That was about naturopathic remedies," he tells me. "It's like homeopathic. I'm going to send my check." He smiles. "He wants me to write out the history of this whole thing, any ideas I have about it."

In the four years since Andy's apparently permanent head-ache, flushing, and body pain began, he has become an anthropologist of alternative medicine. Traditional medicine, too. After innumerable blood tests, a CAT scan, a brain scan, a spinal series, and dozens of other conventional diagnostic procedures, Western medicine has offered him one thing that helps: ibuprofen every three hours. He also searches.

"It's not that I believe there's going to be a cure anymore, but I believe in the process, and I try to enjoy it. I can either bemoan it or make the best of it. So I enjoy meeting these people." Homeopathic practitioners. Naturopaths. Psychic healers. Practitioners of acupuncture, radionics, medical clairvoyance. "Why not? If you get all wrapped up in it, believe in it, you're going to be disappointed, but I'm just finding it fun, for the most part."

It's bad enough to have been visited by the illness. Is it worse to make ourselves vulnerable to quacks? Andy doesn't worry about quacks, partly, I suppose, because he cultivates an attitude of detachment that protects him from abuse. I suspect that if he saw someone who turned out to be an undeniable quack, Andy would respond with curiosity: How interesting! I've never met a real quack before! As it is, he says: "All of them—surgeons to channelers of earth angels that come down and assail your body—are good people. They believe in what they're doing, and I know that every one of these things has helped somebody. Not me. But I've not met one quack."

I, however, am more skeptical. After months and months of illness, I finally gave in to my friends and consulted one not very alternative healer, a homeopathic practitioner with an M.D. from a prestigious university and impeccable mainstream credentials. Homeopathy helped me not at all. Ellen sounds even more conservative than I do. When I ask whether she's tried any alternative remedies, she almost apologizes: "Both my parents are scientists, so I'm into Western medicine."

Ellen and I are at one end of a continuum, Andy at the other end. Ellen waits, as I waited, for Western medicine to help. Just as Andy searches anywhere and everywhere for a cure, a remedy, I searched for a familiar diagnosis, a label that would, I hoped, carry with it a prescription for the right pill, the elusive magic bullet. In the meantime, Western medicine did not tell me to take two aspirin and call in the morning. What a doctor actually said was: "Take *lots* of aspirin and come back in two months." I left the doctor's office and cried. Andy searches. He believes in the process. My process was the search for a diagnosis. So is Erik's. I don't believe in radionics or medical clairvoyance, but I've learned to believe in the search.

ALTERNATIVE REMEDIES CAN
BE DANGEROUS

Not everyone who tries out a non-traditional therapy has a bad experience. But Jean and Mia, her daughter, did. Mia spent the summer before she started college as a camp counselor. Like many other eighteen-year-olds, she got mono. Although she was still unwell in the fall, she started college. She stayed unwell. Eleven doctors and one-and-a-half years later, she was given the diagnosis of chronic Epstein-Barr virus syndrome. Now, six years after her illness began, she is told that she has chronic fatigue syndrome. In her desperate efforts to find something to relieve her daughter's pain and illness, Jean has read, I believe, everything written about the illness and has made sure that Mia receives any treatment that looks promising. Unlike Andy, Jean and Mia have followed medical research, not channelers of earth angels.

Avoiding the psychic fringe didn't protect Jean and Mia from an M.D. in a distant state who billed himself as an environmental allergist. In retrospect, Jean realizes that she should have been suspicious from the start: when she first made Mia's appointment at the doctor's clinic, she was required to send $500 up front. She was told that the treatment would include drops placed under Mia's tongue, and she was assured that if Mia had any negative reaction to the drops, the doctor would be on hand with an antidote. When Jean and Mia kept the appointment, Mia was given the drops and became acutely ill. She was given an antidote. It did nothing. The doctor was not at the clinic. No nurses were there. Indeed, the only people Jean and Mia saw were "testers," people with no medical credentials. Jean eventually managed to see the doctor for ten minutes. He evidenced no alarm at Mia's response to the treatment.

"I can cure her," he assured Jean. "I've cured many patients with multiple sclerosis. I can cure cancer. It's all allergies."

Furious, Jean got up to leave. In parting, the doctor told her that there would be no charge for this consultation. Actually, he sent her a bill for $230. She did not pay it.

"I kick myself for being so stupid," Jean tells me. "That's what happens when you get desperate."

Alison had similar experiences with alternative medicine: one treatment actually caused harm; the others did nothing.

"I couldn't get rid of the flu," Alison says. "I was treated by a holistic doctor who gave me an excess dosage of vitamin A. I got real ill and lost all my hair. I eventually sued him and won the suit." Several years later, recovered from the vitamin A toxicity, she once again came down with an unshakable flu. The doctor she consulted suggested first that she try meditation. Next, "the doctor sent me to an acupuncturist—I'd already seen one—and it did absolutely nothing for me. So I sat down with the acupuncturist and said that maybe I needed a nutritionist." Her doctor also treated her with injections of vitamin C. "I also tried homeopathy. The process was intriguing but one day I found myself dropping all the little white pills all over the bedroom floor. I thought, nothing is happening here. Nothing changed. Nothing ever changed. I went back a couple of times believing that it should change. It didn't seem to bother him that nothing changed."

HERBAL ISN'T ALWAYS SAFE

If you don't need a prescription, it must be safe, right? Especially if you buy it at the health food store.

Pushing her shopping cart through her local whole foods store one day, Norma encountered a salesperson handing out free samples of a Chinese herbal remedy intended to help people suffering from low energy. "Usually, I will not experiment with these things," Norma explains. That day, her energy was so low that she made an exception to her policy. "It was some form of speed, much worse than caffeine!" she reports. "I knew I'd pay for it later. It was amphetamine with a Chinese fancy name. 'Natural and herbal' doesn't mean it's not going to be harmful."

ALTERNATIVE TREATMENTS CAN
BE EXPENSIVE

For $1,800, Andy participated in a program to have all the metal removed from his head. Andy knew what he was in for. He could afford the treatment. He is committed to trying virtually anything, and, given that commitment, the program made sense.

For Greg, even more than for Andy, an expensive treatment is well worth the cost because Greg feels profoundly helped by a therapy compatible with his understanding of his illness. Since Greg understands his illness as an immune system dysfunction that makes him hypersensitive to a wide variety of substances, including viruses, bacteria, common allergens, and substances to which most people are not allergic, he speaks about his neutralizing treatment with his doctor as a joint effort, as something "we" do. To see his doctor, he must drive about forty miles each way.

"When I go up, I typically spend a day there," Greg says.

"How often do you see him?" I ask.

"Once every three to six weeks," Greg tells me. "It's a nuisance, and it's expensive. I figure about three grand a year, between me and the insurance company. On the other hand, I wasn't functioning before, and I hadn't been functioning for some time before I came to him, so it's worth the money."

For Greg, the treatment clearly is worth the money: although his illness continues to impose some limitations, he now works full time, participates in family activities, and otherwise lives a rich life again. "There are people who cannot believe that neutralizing works," he admits, "and that's fine. It can all be placebo as far as I'm concerned. All I know is that I've been back to work for three years." Clearly, Greg has found the right doctor and the right treatment for him. Unfortunately, expense alone does not guarantee either.

Jean's research led her to an experimental program in which she herself served as a donor for her daughter: leukocytes from Jean's blood were processed and then injected in her daughter. The basic idea of this transfer factor treatment is that a healthy person living in close contact with a chronic fatigue syndrome patient is exposed to the illness yet stays well; in effect, what is donated is what enables the donor to stay well. The cost of the program was $5,000 for the first year, and the treatment also required Jean to pay the cost of travel to a distant city as well as hotel and restaurant costs. Jean arranged to pay only half the usual fee for the program, and, after considerable difficulty, arranged to have her insurance company pay for her own medical expenses, but not Mia's. Jean feels that the treatment did benefit Mia. "But," Jean tells me, "you can't donate too often." Consequently, the program refused to let Jean continue to serve as a donor and found an outside donor for Mia, someone also in contact with a CFS patient. "It didn't work," Jean says. "It made her much worse. She was in great pain."

THE UNAPPROVED
MEDICATION ALTERNATIVE

People who decide to pursue non-traditional therapies have many reasons for doing so, but one of the most common ones is frustration with the rate at which new medications and new methods find their way into mainstream medical practice. One complaint of those on the straight experimental route is that funded research studies provide treatments to very small numbers of people. Another is that many drugs reputed to have the potential to help are not available in this country because they lack FDA (Food and Drug Administration) approval. Solution? Get them anyway. An example is isoprinosine, a drug without FDA approval that is supposed to benefit the immune system. Like certain other drugs, it enters this country through Mexico and costs a good deal more here than in its homeland.

Doctors treating CFS patients should bear in mind that isoprinosine is easy to get. One person told me that she'd obtained isoprinosine, tried some, found that it didn't help, then sold the rest to another person with CFS. Doctors uncomfortable prescribing anything at all for patients with a mysterious illness must realize that for many such patients, the easy alternative to prescribed medication is not over-the-counter medication but under-the-counter medication.

UNCERTAIN RESULTS

"I went to see a homeopathic doctor," Leah says. "He gave me these remedies, and my feeling better sometimes seemed to coincide with taking them. The problem with this illness is, because it's up and down, there's no way to know whether something that's done actually helps or whether it's a random association."

As uncertain as the results from any particular alternative remedy may be, however, responses to traditional medications are also difficult to judge. CFS is so mysterious in its comings and goings that it can be hard to tell for sure what effect, if any, a treatment is having.

MEDITATION AND COUNSELING

"There really is no cure," Jean tells me, "and there's not going to be one until they find out the cause."

Many who share Jean's view still continue, as she does for her daughter, to seek help: help for particular symptoms, some amelioration of the overall feeling of being unwell.

Kay, even more than Jean, has sought help primarily in the world of traditional medicine. She hasn't researched any experimental treatments, visited clinics in distant cities, or participated in studies of new drugs. "In the past two years, I've had everything suggested to me from acupuncture to vitamin C intravenously. I went to a nutritionist who recommended all this stuff that I never did. It involved taking all these nutritional supplements, over twenty-four pills a day. It was this whole regimen, and it was very expensive. I checked it out with my internist, and she said that she thought stuff like that really didn't help."

Kay did try, however, two things suggested at one time or another to almost everyone with a chronic fatigue illness: she went to a mind-body clinic to learn meditation. And she went to a psychiatrist.

"I found," Kay says, "that I *couldn't* meditate. I'd get all anxious, and I couldn't do it. So it turned out to be a fairly negative experience because I found out, now, on top of everything else, that I can't even meditate!"

Alison's experience was similar: "It was work. I *could* not meditate. The sensations in my body were so bizarre. And I'd always had a sense of my body being relaxed or strong, so I was dealing with anguish about that." Just what you need when you are ill: an increased sense of incompetence.

For many people with a chronic fatigue illness, the initial and sometimes prolonged search for medical help means repeated suggestions from general practitioners, internists, and specialists to see a psychiatrist. To many, such a suggestion sounds like an insult, an unwelcome accusation of hypochondriacal mental illness, more evidence of not being taken seriously: go have your head examined! That was not Kay's attitude in seeking therapy. "All the people who suggest that psychotherapy is going to make this go away are wrong. I'm a real believer in psychotherapy as something helpful to people, but it doesn't make this go away." To Kay, therapy did offer something valuable, however—help in learning to cope more effectively with her illness.

DO ALTERNATIVE TREATMENTS
EVER WORK?

Despite the negative experiences of many of the people with whom I spoke, others, like Greg, have found relief and even health through non-traditional approaches.

Maya tells me that the most helpful practitioners she encountered were neither traditional doctors, nor CFS experts, nor any other doctors, but "strange people with strange backgrounds." Indeed, the most helpful, she says, was an eccentric homeopathic practitioner who had dropped out of medical school and who maintained a tumble-down office filled with odd bottles and jars. Before she was diagnosed with Lyme disease, he prescribed an herbal tea "that *really* helped. Month to month, I started to feel better. The trend was in the right direction." As Maya stresses to me, a welcome advantage of the non-traditional practitioners she consulted was cost. The EBV experts she'd been seeing were expensive: She was paying $200 for each office visit. She was given EBV tests every month at $250 per test. In contrast, the eccentric homeopath charged her $30 a visit, and he helped. Diagnosed with Lyme disease and treated with the antibiotics essential to prevent the neurologic, heart, head, and joint abnormalities caused by Lyme disease, Maya did not experience a restoration of energy and health but found herbal teas, dietary changes, and other holistic remedies all helpful in restoring energy.

Ginny has no interest in alternative treatments. For several years, however, a friend had been telling her about bee pollen. "It's supposed to build the immune system, help fight viruses, strep. I was skeptical. I didn't even believe in vitamins," Ginny says. She did notice, though, that her friend and her friend's family seemed to be remarkably healthy. The friend kept urging her to try the bee pollen. "After two years, I couldn't think of any reason to put it off. I went on it. Then when I stopped for four or five days, I got a sinus infection." She started taking it again and started to get better. Furthermore, she noticed to her surprise that her hands, previously cracked and bleeding, were healing. "I thought, wait a minute! In spite of myself, I was starting to feel a little better." Nine months after she began to take the remedy in which she did not believe, she describes herself as "pretty good." She says: "Sometimes I get that old feeling, but I rest and feel better." Using almost the same words Greg uses in talking about neutralizing, she tells me, "If it's a placebo effect, I don't care."

DISCOMFORT WITH ALTERNATIVE REMEDIES

Ellen, who shares what many of my friends called my hide-bound Western-scientific attitudes, limited her explorations to mainstream medicine. Marna, too, tried an alternative only when "fed up with Western medicine." Those of us who avoid the alternatives seem to me to share some characteristics beyond what strikes others as narrow-mindedness.

First, as we're apt to say, we're not alternative types. Second, we seem to lack a coherent concept of what's making us sick. We tend, as Marna says, to be people who "don't think the diagnosis means anything." Fed up, desperate, eager to silence the friends urging us to try the alternatives, we select the most mainstream, least alternative alternatives. We see respectable homeopathic M.D.'s. We try acupuncture. Overall, however, if a treatment doesn't make sense to us, we won't try it, and since the illness doesn't make sense to us, treatments don't either.

A variation of this occurs when a person trusts a doctor who has little faith in finding effective remedies, especially in alternative healing systems. Kay, for instance, tells me, "My doctor is fairly conservative. Her attitude is pretty much, try it if you want to, but I don't really believe it's going to help. Hearing that doesn't inspire me to go off and try stuff."

If you feel more comfortable with alternative remedies than do Ellen or Kay or I—if you are closer to Andy's end of the spectrum of attitudes on this subject than to ours, by all means pursue non-traditional approaches. As Jean and Mia, Alison, and Norma found out, alternative treatments may pose risks to your health and finances. On the other hand, some of these treatments seem to help some people. Above all else, the process of searching for something, no matter what, benefits virtually everyone.

8

Support Groups and Antidepressants

THE SEARCH FOR SOMETHING
THAT HELPS

Itt has made such a difference!"

Many people say it, and I wish that I, in turn, could report that what makes a difference is always amitriptyline, a support group, a macrobiotic diet, or some other replicable thing or combination of things. For Andy, two things make a difference: first, ibuprofen, and, second, the process of searching for a cure. For a few people, the search for one specific remedy that makes a big difference has led to a cure or a major lessening of symptoms. For others, amelioration sometimes just happens. It is as mysterious as falling ill was in the first place.

"How did you get better?" I ask Kay, who is better than she was, though not all better.

"God knows," she answers. "How did I get sick?"

For most people, however, what makes a difference is neither a specific remedy that vanquishes symptoms nor is it the passage of time or the intervention of mysterious good luck. Rather, it is help in managing the illness that comes from someone, somewhere: The right doctor. The right support group. The right therapist. Yourself.

USING EXISTING NETWORKS

Kay takes for granted neither her friends nor her employer. "My friends were wonderful." She says of her company, "It's a wonderful place to work." What she does perhaps take for granted is her own skill in using the help her friends and employer have provided. When Kay was acutely ill, her friends helped. When she was in the hospital, they visited her. "They volunteered," she says, but later she tells me, "I don't have frivolous friendships. I have good friendships. I never felt that I wanted to hide stuff from my friends. You don't want to burden any one of them by accepting too many favors."

In a comparable way, after tremendous resistance to taking time off from a job she loves, Kay finally admitted the need to take advantage of her company's disability policy. "They're known as being a good employer, and I think they are. They do a lot to look out for employees' interests. Their benefits are very good." Obviously, to take advantage of the help offered by a good employer requires having a good one. Not everyone does. Even for Kay, obtaining benefits and absenting herself from work were not easy. Nonetheless, it is clear that Kay not only had supportive networks, but knew that she had them and knew how to use them.

Alex's employer, in contrast to Kay's, refused to pay any benefits. "They didn't believe it was a real illness," he says of his chronic fatigue syndrome. He applied for disability benefits under Social Security and was once again denied. Having tried and failed to find help from two existing networks, he mobilized the help of a third: the political connections he had built up through volunteer work in his community. "I made a few phone calls," he says, "and met one person who'd heard of the disease. He put me in touch with a fellow at Social Security who took my case on and got me though it." Although Alex was twice denied benefits under Social Security, he eventually obtained those benefits as well as the benefits his employer had originally denied him. It seems unlikely that he could have done so on his own.

Not everyone has Kay's network of friends or excellent employer. Most of us lack Alex's political connections. Laura, the widowed mother of a young child, found tremendous emotional support and practical help from the members of her church, who took turns shopping and cooking meals for her, but not everyone goes to church, and not everyone's life situation so readily elicits help. Kay, however, could have convinced her friends that she did not need help. Alex could have failed to use his political network. Laura could have prevented the members of her church from assisting her. Not everyone has their networks, of course, but some of us refuse the help available to us.

ORGANIZING

Sometimes the organized network is not waiting out there ready to be mobilized; rather, it is a potential network waiting to be organized. "It was so clear," says Alison, "once the diagnosis [of CEBV] was in, either friends were on the down side and were terrified, or they were saying, 'What can I do?' People who could see through the illness to the person. Basically, I felt like an organizer. The thing I needed most was to have a lot of hugging and to cry, to have people sit with me and let me cry. I needed to be taken out. I found that I really had to say: 'I just need to be sick with someone near me.'"

SUPPORT FROM PETS

My first word was *dog*. My first memory is of dogs. I am not sane on the subject. When my illness started, I had a nine-month-old Alaskan malamute. A young malamute should be running, playing, learning to pull a sled, and taking its first obedience lessons. Mine spent many days in a darkened room. When my family and friends were busy or thoroughly fed up with me and my illness, my dog sat by my bed and rested her paw in my hand. Whenever possible, I walked her, played with her, and trained her. It was not always possible. I swore that if I ever recovered, I would make those months up to her. I have.

Until I talked with Alex, I imagined that finding such emotional support from a dog was merely one more instance of my lunacy on the subject. "Thank God for my animals," Alex says of a menagerie that includes two Clumber spaniels and a cat. "They were just there. They were with me. It seemed like everyone else in the world had run off."

FINDING THE RIGHT DOCTOR

"It took me a year to find a doctor who understands this illness," Roseanne says. "I have a superb doctor now. It's made a world of difference, psychologically."

Alex has had the same doctor for twenty years. "My doctor is fabulous," he says. "We have quite a rapport. We've joined forces and hung in there together."

Greg believes in his doctor's treatment and in his doctor. "He's an old-style doctor," Greg says. "He learned, like all M.D.'s, to act big, important. But also, somewhere along the line, he learned another method of treating people."

Roseanne's doctor, superb for her, might not be right for Greg, and Greg's might not be right for Roseanne, Meg, or me. Some people do find the right doctors for them, and when that perfect match occurs, it makes one of the biggest differences. It may not be worth the energy to search for the perfect doctor, but I believe that in some circumstances, we must summon the energy to rid ourselves of doctors who are almost as burdensome as our illnesses. As Kay says: "Where I draw the line is with physicians who do not listen and who simply discount what they can't see. Because they don't know, it doesn't exist. I have no sympathy for that attitude."

THE RIGHT MEDICATION

There is no evidence that any medication cures chronic fatigue syndrome. Also, some people with chronic fatigue illnesses are given prescription drugs that, alone or in combination, may cause or exacerbate the symptoms of the illness; and prescription drugs that may entail physical and psychological dependence. Nevertheless, prescription drugs are often a part of the treatment, though not the cure, for CFS.

Can prescribed medication make a difference? For some people, yes. A big difference. When that was the case for the people who talked with me—no scientific sample—the biggest help came from low doses of tricyclic antidepressants.

Alex had had a pattern of disturbed sleep. In some phases of his illness, he would sleep for eighteen hours a day. For four or five days, he would then be unable to sleep at all. His doctor prescribed ten milligrams a day of doxepin. Alex says that "it flattened me." He adds: "But, it helped." Despite feeling flattened, he continued taking it, and after a week, "the heavy effects left." He continues to take ten milligrams of doxepin every evening. "I can count on six or seven hours of good sleep. It's the only thing that's helped."

When Greg returned to work after a six-month absence, his company's medical department suggested that he see a psychiatrist, and Greg complied. Although the psychiatrist said that he saw no reason for Greg to be in psychotherapy, he suggested that imipramine, a tricyclic antidepressant, might be worth a try. Like many people with chronic fatigue syndrome, Greg finds himself much more sensitive to drugs than most other people. Besides, he trusts his own doctor and wanted his advice about dosage. The psychiatrist originally suggested that Greg work up to 150 milligrams a day. Greg consulted his own doctor. "We decided I'd start with five," Greg says. "God, slowly the depression eased. I'm now taking between twenty and thirty milligrams. It made it so much easier to cope at work."

I, however, was not as fortunate. When I first heard the theory that CEBV or chronic fatigue syndrome impedes restful sleep and that amitriptyline helps to induce sound sleep, it seemed like a terrific idea, even though I resisted those diagnoses. I was sleeping, but I was certainly not sleeping restfully. If only I could sleep very deeply, maybe I would recover, I thought. My doctor, too, had heard that very small doses of amitriptyline were being prescribed for illnesses like mine, and she, too, thought it was worth a try. At eight o'clock in the evening, I took one ten-milligram tablet of amitriptyline. The tablets don't come any smaller; the usual dosage is 75 to 150 milligrams a day. At eight o'clock the next morning I emerged from sleep in a state of groggy semi-consciousness, stupefied and miserable. At one o'clock that afternoon, I dragged myself out of bed, took a hot shower, drank two cups of strong coffee, and swore never again to take amitriptyline. Ginny's experience was like mine. Maybe she and I, like Alex, should have continued taking the drug until the side effects wore off, but I'm not sure that in a week there would have been anything left of me to benefit.

Marna *has* benefited, however. She takes ten milligrams of amitriptyline at bedtime. "It *helps!*" she says, although she finds that the drug makes it hard for her to get up in the morning and wonders whether she now takes it "because of superstition." Wary of drugs, she nonetheless takes meclizine for vertigo and alprazolam for anxiety when she needs the help they provide. "I'm careful," she says.

EXPERT BACK-UP

So you've met the right doctor, but he's an expert on chronic fatigue syndrome with 40,000 referrals a year, and, besides, your health maintenance organization won't pay for you to see him anyway. People fortunate enough to find the right expert sometimes manage to get a single appointment or one visit a year. Ginny, Don, and Leah, who belong to health maintenance organizations, managed to see such experts. As Leah suggests, such an expert is most helpful as a back-up in dealing with a skeptical regular doctor when the expert is highly regarded in the mainstream medical community: the expert "did confirm to everybody's satisfaction that I do indeed have this illness, and they believe him because he's trained all of them," Leah explains. Before joining a health maintenance organization, Ellen saw a highly esteemed expert on chronic fatigue syndrome. When a change in the medical insurance available to her made it necessary to switch to the health maintenance organization, the expert, whom she was reluctant to leave ("He was my lifeline, the only one who understood"), referred her to a doctor at the HMO, and has continued to serve as a consultant.

Susan Conant

PSYCHOTHERAPY

When people find the right medication, it helps a lot. Similarly, when people find the right therapist, therapy makes a big difference. Do we, as our critics suggest we should, discover that the illness is, after all, only in our heads? That we are making ourselves sick? On the contrary, one way in which therapy can help tremendously is to let us differentiate clearly enough between ourselves and our illnesses to recognize our illnesses for what they are. "Therapy helped me to realize it *was* physical," Marna says. Her therapist "validated the fact that it was physical, that I wasn't crazy."

Whether or not we have already had that realization and validation, therapy can also help us, as it has Ellen, to manage our illnesses and our changed lives. In the acute phases of illness, therapy can offer one relationship that requires no pretense of great physical or mental health. Kay says of one phase of her illness: "I was so sick that I really couldn't deal with anything. I was seeing a psychiatrist twice a week, and it was all I could do to get myself there. I spent all my time in her office crying and just being a mess."

For Alison, who found efforts to meditate anything but relaxing, a therapist's use of hypnosis offered a helpful alternative. "In therapy, the reason for doing the hypnosis was that I needed to tune out all these noises going on inside me, especially the pain in my head and ears, and to re-experience the pain as relaxation, which is really hard to do. It was called 'plunging into pain' in some book I read, but for me, it was guiding myself into the pain, not being scared of it. And it really, really helped. I did hypnosis with my therapist a couple of times, and we put it on tape. Now I can do it at home, too. It's hard work for me, but it made a huge difference."

Wendy initially resisted the idea of therapy: "I was furious at the entire medical profession. All they had told me was that I was crazy." To go to a therapist, it seemed, was "an admission that they were right." She went to a therapist only because her sister all but forced her to do so. "I remember thinking when I first started that this was the most ridiculous, futile thing. It was the stupidest thing I could do: you go into therapy with marriage problems, and you can figure out your marriage problems, or you can divorce the guy, or

LIVING WITH CHRONIC FATIGUE

you can work it out. Or you go in with job problems, and you can change jobs. But you can't go to therapy to get better and go on with your life! So why was I sitting in this guy's office? He wasn't going to do any kind of intervention that was really going to do anything."

"But," she adds, "I'm delighted to say that I was wrong. I think I have become physically much better through psychotherapy. It didn't cure me, but, if nothing else, you don't complicate your illness by becoming so overengaged with the disease that it really wins. I am quite certain that when I started therapy, I was as profoundly unhappy as I'd ever been in my life. I have to say that I'm reasonably happy at this point. Happy. And sick."

But therapy is not always helpful. Alex, who has an excellent 20-year relationship with his doctor, took seriously his doctor's suggestion that he talk to a psychiatrist about issues in his life. After six sessions, the psychiatrist analyzed a number of Alex's physical symptoms as representations of events in his early childhood. "I missed my father and was reverting to my childhood," Alex says. "I walked out."

SUPPORT GROUPS AND ORGANIZATIONS

The organizations created and run by and for people with CEBV, CFS, or CFIDS—the names have changed over the years—offer several distinct kinds of help. Local support groups, as the name suggests, are intended to provide personal support to individuals mainly by bringing together individuals and families who share the illness. Local, state, and national organizations not only sponsor support groups but also have educational and political aims. They distribute educational information about the illness to people who have it, to the general public, and to policy makers whose decisions influence the lives of people with the illness. These organizations also work directly to persuade legislators and others to increase the funding for research on the illness and to make financial support available to people too ill to work.

For Don, a support group meant "relief at hearing similar experiences," the confirmation that there was "an objective reality to it." As other people with CFS have said, there was validation in discovering that "you're not the only one."

"It was an eye-opener," Greg says of his first group. "We weren't alone any more."

"I was seeking compassion and support," Ellen says. "No one could really understand it, so it was good to find the group."

Alex, one of the founders of the support group in his town, continues to lead the group. As group leader, he takes an active role. It was he who arranged to have the group meet in his church. Once or twice a month, between meetings, he calls all of the members of his group. Convinced that support groups function best when they serve families rather than individuals, he works to involve spouses. "It's been phenomenal," he says. "I've seen people who are so shattered be able to pull together. Husbands and wives start to talk again. We all feel so much a part of it. We've got something special."

When Group Support Fails

Unfortunately, Alex is right in feeling that his group is unusual. Some groups encounter problems so severe that they flounder and eventually end. Others meet the needs of some members, but find that other potential members never attend or drop out after a few meetings. Furthermore, support groups are not for everyone. Sometimes there is a simple explanation of why someone does not attend meetings: Roseanne has never been to a group because she is too tired and sick to go. "It's one more thing," she says. "If it's optional, forget it."

Sometimes, however, people attend a meeting or two and drop out. Although contact with others who share the illness is supposed to offer the relief and support that Don and Alex find, groups do not always work as they are supposed to. "There are many people there sicker than you," Marna says. "It's really depressing. I ran out of there and went home and went to bed." In particular, a group may succeed so well in emphasizing the similarity of people's experiences and symptoms that it may fail to support a person whose experience of illness differs from the group norms and definitions.

LIVING WITH CHRONIC FATIGUE

"I've never had swollen glands," Marna says. The group members, however, said, "Oh, you will!"

Some of the problems that support groups encounter are attributable to the diversity of the needs the groups try to meet, others to a lack of trained leadership. "I ran support groups for a while," someone told me. "It is tremendously difficult to do the little local support groups. There are always new patients. They always want things answered that old patients don't want to hear about. The old patients need to spend more time focusing on how to make the world worthwhile and productive. And the support group leadership. We've tried to delegate it to patients, and you can do that if they're trained, but we've all had the experience of trying to run support group meetings and knowing how limited we are."

Kay depicts what can happen without trained leadership: "It didn't have any structure to it at all. It was a bunch of people sitting around saying, 'Oh, I tried this, I tried that.' It wasn't supportive. It wasn't like people were really getting to know each other."

Why is the leadership untrained? First, there is no money to pay for professional group leadership, supervision, or consultation. For example, the income of the Massachusetts CFIDS Association consists almost exclusively of membership dues, $15 a year from each member, which must pay for all of the association's activities, not just small groups. Second, because associations and groups are run almost solely by volunteers, most of whom are ill, the number of potential volunteer leaders with appropriate professional training who have the time and energy to run a group is minuscule. On the principle of deleting optional activities, many sick people drop all volunteer work. For many, continuing to work is so important that they follow the familiar pattern of working, sleeping, working, sleeping, with no time in between. Marna, for example, has training appropriate for leading a group, but has worked throughout most of her illness and is now actively job hunting. At some point, she says, she would like to start her own support group, but now is not the time.

A final reason that some people avoid support groups and, indeed, avoid active participation in CFS associations is a phenomenon Leah described. Having joined the state association, she attended several presentations about the illness. "I didn't much want to have anything to do with the other people in the room. I stayed for the discussion groups the first few times, and it was clear to me that the larger group there was made up of people like me who'd just been diagnosed and were seeking information. The others were people who had been sick for a long time and who carried this as a major piece of their identity and who didn't seem to be upset anymore about being sick. They accepted being sick as a way of life. And I knew for sure that I never wanted to do that. Frankly, with limited energy, I'd rather spend it doing something that's part of a regular life instead of part of a sickness life. Information? Fine. Identity? No, thank you."

A related difficulty that a few people reported encountering at lectures and other large meetings and in some other contacts with associations was what Roseanne calls "exclusivity." "They almost ask for your EBV titers, and they want your doctor's name to make sure it's one they like." Leah, who perceives the same defensiveness, explains it this way: "This illness involves a long period of being misunderstood. I see it as a reaction to something that happened before."

NATIONAL AND LOCAL ORGANIZATIONS

Whereas support groups received mixed reviews, efforts to educate and inform people about their illnesses and to reach out to those who do not attend groups or meetings are almost unequivocally successful and universally appreciated. Indeed, staying informed is so helpful that the next chapter of this book consists of a guide to resources, many of which would be unavailable without the help of national and local organizations.

Roseanne, too ill to go to any meetings, nonetheless belongs to an association, borrows tapes of educational lectures through its by-mail lending service, and receives its newsletter, which she finds very helpful. "Especially the personal articles," she says. "I pick up an article, and I feel like I wrote it. I'm not alone!"

Most medical articles, of course, are published in journals unavailable in local public libraries. Without the services of associations, most such articles would be unavailable to the people with the illnesses on which the articles focus. National organizations, how-ever, make it possible to say routinely, as many people did, "I wrote away for the article on. . . ." Providing access to these articles is a great service.

For many people, one valuable function the associations have served is to inform both doctors and patients that these illnesses exist. People described first learning about the CEBV syndrome or CFS from a television show, magazine story, or newspaper report that focused on a national organization. "There was all this stuff about Epstein-Barr in the news," Kay says. "I started to read about it, and I thought: I have it. I just knew." Without national organiza-tions, there would have been few such stories, and many people would have struggled alone in the belief that they were the only people ever visited by such an illness.

HELPING OTHERS

Leading support groups, organizing and running associations, and taking part in political activities related to the illness are, for some people, a way of fighting back. That's not quite what they are for Alex. Besides leading a local support group, he participates in statewide meetings and other efforts aimed at social and legislative change. "Getting active saved my life," he says. One of the few people who spoke directly to me about finding help through reli-gious beliefs, Alex says, "God has given me this attitude: Take this, and make what you can of it. When people understand that they're not alone, they start rebuilding everything they've lost, self-esteem, everything. It's in giving that we receive."

CARING FOR YOURSELF

"For a long-term illness," says Andy, "the only way to treat yourself is to treat yourself well. The quality of your life has got to become paramount." Sometimes in search of cures or remedies, sometimes in search of an improvement in the quality of their lives, people come across things that do not affect the illness but that do help because they feel good and because they counter the sense of being worthless and hence undeserving.

Finally fed up with Western medicine, Marna went for acupuncture for a few months. "It did nothing," she says. She then tried massage, which she continues although it is equally ineffective against her illness. "It's a treat I give myself. It feels much better than acupuncture."

In a somewhat similar way, Kay has taken up Tai Chi. "I get little or no exercise, which is bad, and I figure it's a little exercise, but it's not like aerobics or something strenuous. It's something I *can* do. Once I started it, I really liked it. It feels like a nice thing to be doing for myself."

DEVISING A PROGRAM

"The best I'm doing is managing this illness," Don says as if that weren't a remarkable achievement. Leah speaks not only of managing the illness but of having decided to do so. "When I decided to manage the illness," she says, "I knew that nothing from the outside was going to help."

Of what does management consist? Certainly not of trying to become the wonderful manager whose life doesn't change because of a mere illness. People who described managing the illness have worked out individual multi-component programs that work for them. These programs do not cure the illness, and they do not work quickly. But in the long run, they help.

For Ellen and Leah, who don't share my ambivalent feelings about the subject, one important component is minimizing stress. "I'd read that once you had this illness," Leah says, "any stress or any physiological response could kick you into relapse. I made a decision that I was not going to experience any emotional upset, and, on the whole, I kept it." Everyone rests. For Leah, Don, and others, another component is exercise at a monitored and regulated level. His doctor's program, in combination with other efforts, works for Greg: neutralizing treatments, vitamin supplements, and the strict regulation of diet to exclude junk food, including sugar. "It all adds up," Greg says in emphasizing, as do others, that "there isn't any one answer."

HEALING OURSELVES

If we can help ourselves, can't we go all the way and heal ourselves, too? Some books and theories suggest we can.

"I highly object to the attitude that if you're only an exceptional patient, you can cure cancer," says Andy. "What about the people who die? Were they all bad patients? We're all going to die. We die because we're bad? We get sick because we're bad or we're doing something wrong? And the superior people are well. I think that's a myth. It's unhelpful to the people who are feeling well and the people who are feeling sick. It feeds the illusion to those people who are feeling well that they're well because they're well put together. And it feeds the self-hatred of the people who are not feeling well. It's blaming the victim."

I agree. So does Marna. She says, "There's a fine line between blame and responsibility." Kay agrees: "Our society has gone a little overboard about people's ability to heal themselves. This disease has become an example of a place where you should be able to do that. It used to be presumed that you had chemotherapy if you had cancer. Now there's a lot of research to suggest that there are other things to do. But that gets misinterpreted, overplayed to the point that it's a blaming-the-victim type of thing, or it feels that way. People feel that you *should* be able to make yourself better. I think it's insidious because you start to believe that yourself: What's wrong with me? Why did I get this in the first place?"

Can we heal ourselves? I found the injunction so enraging that I fooled myself into thinking that everyone would agree. Roseanne does not. "I sometimes wonder if I'm not allowing myself to heal fully," she says. It is clear, however, that she views self-healing as a source of hope, not blame, and that she views it, as she said repeatedly, as "theoretical." Furthermore, unlike most of us, she accepts with apparent equanimity the notion that only the exceptional heal themselves: "Maybe some people have more psychological hardware than I do," she says. In her voice I hear none of the anger that fills Andy's, Marna's, Kay's, and mine when we talk about the idea that we could or should heal ourselves.

Can we heal ourselves? The belief in self-healing makes a difference to Roseanne. It helps her. And the rest of us? For most of us, encountering in others the belief that we could or should heal ourselves makes a difference, too. It hurts.

FINDING SOMETHING THAT HELPS

This disagreement over the theory of self-healing perfectly illustrates how important it is for you to decide for yourself what *you* think makes a big difference. Learning about the experiences of other chronically ill people can be enormously valuable in making you realize you are not alone and in giving you new ideas for possible treatments and ways to cope. But only you can decide what helps you feel better, both physically and psychologically.

What counts most, though, is not *what* you decide but *that* you decide for yourself.

9

Books, Newsletters, and Audiotapes:

LEARNING ABOUT CFS

Don't read about it," an internist recently told Alison. "The more you do, the worse you'll feel."

Nonsense. Leah and I went through phases of reading everything we could find, yet her illness is now in remission, and I've recovered. For someone with CFS, Roseanne does relatively little technical reading, yet she's still sick. Meg read little about illness and has fully recovered from whatever mysterious thing she had. Reading does not keep you ill. It keeps you informed.

"I have a folder," Kay tells me. We exchange glances. We smile. I know just what her folder looks like, and I know what's in it. "There's no point in my running back and forth to doctors all the time," Kay says. "The articles may not be very uplifting because there's not a lot of good news, but I'd rather know than not know."

"I used to read anything I could get," Don tells me. He went to a medical library to look up technical articles in journals. Leah wrote away for what she calls "those dreadful medical articles." Some of us pass copies of articles along to our doctors. Others receive them from their doctors. When Laura's doctor diagnosed her CEBV, the illness was little known. To help her understand it, he gave her copies of medical articles. Meg was amused and cheered when her father sent her dozens of clippings from magazines and newspapers and photocopies of pages from medical dictionaries and medical books. She wasn't interested in reading the clippings and photocopies, but she appreciated her father's efforts. "He was trying," she says.

OBTAINING MATERIALS

Some of the books mentioned here are available in public libraries. If your local library does not have a book you particularly want, you might ask whether the book is available through an inter-library loan or you might ask to have the book ordered. *The Merck Manual* and other reference books are usually kept in a library's reference room and usually do not circulate.

Manuals, booklets, and such are not apt to be in public libraries, but many local CFS associations and support groups maintain lending libraries through which you may borrow these materials. If you borrow by mail, there is usually a small fee for postage and handling. If you decide to order by mail, bear in mind that addresses and prices may change, so it is a good idea to write for information before mailing a check.

MATERIALS AVAILABLE FROM ASSOCIATIONS

Three national CFS/CFIDS associations provide information about the illness: the CFIDS Society (formerly the National CEBV Association), in Portland, Oregon; the National Chronic Fatigue Syndrome Association, in Kansas City; and the CFIDS Association, in Charlotte, North Carolina. A new umbrella organization, the United Federation of CFS/CFIDS/CEBV Organizations, coordinates the effort of the three groups, which specialize in providing different kinds of information.

The CFIDS Society
P.O. Box 230108
Portland, Oregon 97223

The Chronic Fatigue Immune Dysfunction Syndrome Society distributes basic information about CFIDS, but it is best known as a convenient source of otherwise almost inaccessible journal articles about the illness. Your local library doesn't have *The Scandinavian Journal of Immunology?* Not even *The New England Journal of Medicine?* Through the CFIDS Society, you'll be able to order a reprint of practically any article ever published that has anything to do with the illness, pamphlets on Social Security disability benefits, tapes of CFS/CFIDS conferences, and even transcripts of some conferences.

National CFS Association
12106 East 54th Terrace
Kansas City, Missouri 64133

or

919 Scott Avenue
Kansas City, Kansas 66105

The National Chronic Fatigue Syndrome Association distributes a series of brochures and information packets and produces an excellent newsletter. Particularly laudable is this group's avoidance of a commitment to any particular hypothesis about what causes the syndrome. A pamphlet called "Social Security Disability Benefits Information" should provide a good starting point for anyone in need of such benefits. (The initial mailing costs the association $2.00, so if possible, include a check with your request for materials.)

The CFIDS Chronicle
The CFIDS Association
Community Health Services
P.O. Box 220398
Charlotte, North Carolina 28222-0398

The journal of the Chronic Fatigue and Immune Dysfunction Syndrome Association, *The CFIDS Chronicle,* is a must for anyone who wants to stay in touch with medical research and political advocacy related to this illness. If you want the details of all the latest hypotheses about what's making you ill, the results of treatment studies, statements of testimony to Congress, reviews of articles about CFIDS, and lots more, don't miss this journal. Vastly more polished and professional than local newsletters, it still retains some of their personal, on-our-side feeling. One warning: because this journal covers just about all CFIDS developments, it may tell you much more than you want to know.

A GUIDE TO RESEARCH

Many of the articles distributed by the CFIDS Society and other organizations are reports of research. If you have no formal training in research yet want to decode academic papers, understand reports of studies, and otherwise figure out what research means, be sure to read *Summing Up: The Science of Reviewing Research* (1984) by Richard J. Light and David B. Pillemer. It is a practical, readable guide to evaluating research and summarizing research findings.

BOOKS, BOOKLETS, AND MANUALS ON CHRONIC FATIGUE SYNDROME

Chronic Fatigue Syndrome: A Victim's Guide to Understanding, Treating, and Coping With This Debilitating Illness (1989) by Gregg Charles Fisher is a revised and updated edition of *Waiting to Live: The Debilitating Effects of Chronic Epstein-Barr Virus* (1987).

In the winter of 1982, Gregg Fisher was studying to become a minister, and the woman he eventually married was working on a master's degree in counseling and psychology. When both became ill, she was quickly diagnosed with mononucleosis. Although his symptoms were very similar to hers, his blood test for mono was negative. Neither of them recovered from the illness; neither has yet recovered. Both were eventually diagnosed with CEBV.

In both editions of this book, Fisher presents a personal account of his struggle with the illness and information about its diagnosis and treatment. The editions differ mainly in the emphasis on the Epstein-Barr virus. Fisher's presentation of information about the syndrome is clear and comprehensive.

The chapter on diagnosis (Chapter 4 of both editions) seems directed more toward making sure that you receive the diagnosis of CEBV (first edition) or CFS (second edition) than toward making sure that you don't have some other illness.

For Fisher and his wife, the illness has been very debilitating, as the titles of both editions indicate. When they decided to get married, they also applied for disability benefits and have continued to receive disability benefits under Social Security. Chapter 7 (of both editions) includes a description of applying for those benefits that should be helpful to anyone too ill to work.

The chapters on living with CFS describe Fisher's and his wife's experience, together with advice for people with CEBV/CFS and for their families and friends. The descriptions of the symptoms of the illness and the experience of living with those symptoms are detailed.

Fisher portrays what I most feared when I was sick: life transmuted to illness. Even though I read *Waiting To Live* after I had recovered, I nonetheless found it so depressing that I could hardly finish it. Several people told me that they could not finish it. "It was so depressing," Kay says. "These poor people. My heart went out to them. I don't know anyone who's as sick as they are, and they don't seem to be getting better at all." She read about half of the book. "I thought, I don't need to do this."

Some readers with perspectives different from mine find Fisher's writing helpful and even comforting. Don did. Of Fisher and his wife, Don says, "Their experience was similar to mine in terms of having to give things up, get sufficient rest, putting my body first." If you read this book, however, remember two points that receive little mention in it: first, some people recover. Second, the adaptations that Fisher recommends are not the only kinds of adaptations people make to serious chronic illness.

You may or may not want to read Jesse Stoff and Charles Pellegrino's *Chronic Fatigue Syndrome: The Hidden Epidemic* (1988). Jesse Stoff is a physician with training in holistic medicine and homeopathy. He and Pellegrino, a biologist and consultant on spaceflight, were boyhood friends. This book is, first, the story of Stoff's treatment of Pellegrino for an illness they both attribute to the Epstein-Barr virus. Second, despite its title, it is a book about that virus and how to cure illnesses like Pellegrino's. What is this miracle cure? Why didn't we think of it? We did. It consists of a combination of homeopathy, exercise, nutrition, vitamin and mineral supplements, and positive thinking. "I was disgusted," Jean says. "I'm very disgusted with him."

Does Stoff actually claim to cure the illness? He hedges. He admits that no one has discovered a way to eliminate the Epstein-Barr virus from the body.

To a large extent, however, the book is based on the belief in a causal link between the Epstein-Barr virus and chronic fatigue syndrome. If you read only this book, you'd never know that the hypothesis of that causal link has been challenged by many people and discarded by most as an explanation of all or most cases of CFS. Also, the claim of the effectiveness of the treatment is based strictly on the recounting of a few cases, plus Stoff's vague generalizations about his patients. This books offers no evidence from systematic study, never mind evidence from a randomized, controlled trial of this treatment. And the treatment itself is nothing new; parts of it help some of us but not others, sometimes but not always.

Barbara Brooks and Nancy Smith, the authors of *CFIDS: An Owner's Manual* (1988), are friends who share a doctor as well as the illness they call CFIDS. Although this manual gives a brief account of their stories, it consists mainly of advice. Before a visit to any doctor, write down the questions you want to ask. Learn to listen to your body. Concentrate on what you can do instead of on what you can't. Use a light-weight carpet sweeper instead of a big vacuum cleaner. The book consists mainly of these kinds of survival tips and exhortations to develop a positive attitude. (Copies may be ordered by sending a check for $12.95 payable to Barbara Brooks to BBNS, P.O. Box 6456, Silver Spring, Maryland 20906.)

Chronic Fatigue and Immune Dysfunction (Chronic Epstein-Barr Virus) Syndrome: Patient Information, Fourth Edition, compiled and distributed by the Houston CFIDS Support Group, contains much more information about the Epstein-Barr virus than most people will want. Especially for the newly diagnosed, the emphasis on that perhaps irrelevant and certainly boring virus may be confusing. Still, this booklet contains reprints of several informative and important articles as well as copies of several misleading and out-of-date ones. The now-classic "Chronic Fatigue Syndrome: A Working Case Definition" (1988) appears here, as do a number of original first-person accounts and first-person accounts from popular magazines. If you have not read Hillary Johnson's "Journey Into Fear," a two-part article originally published in *Rolling Stone* (1987), this is an easy place to find it. (To order, send $17.50 to The Houston CFIDS Support Group, 8820 Memorial Drive, Houston, Texas 77024.)

John W. Endsley's *Understanding Chronic Fatigue Syndrome: Practical Information for Patients* is a twenty-five page booklet that summarizes information about the illness, Endsley's long personal experience with it, symptoms, possible causes, research findings, treatments, and such. The writing is more succinct yet more detailed and the tone less depressing than in many comparable presentations of information. (To order, send $4.95 plus $1.50 shipping and handling to John Endsley, Department R., 350 Lamplighter Lane, Marietta, Georgia 30067.)

When I ordered *Chronic Fatigue Syndrome: A Personal Diary* (1988), by Arnold H. Goldberg, M.D., I expected a personal narrative about the author's illness. As it turns out, he's perfectly healthy. You're the one who's supposed to keep the diary.

Has your illness been so fascinating that you want to record each shining hour? Alternatively, has it been so imperceptible that you are apt to forget it? If so, this book is for you. It consists of a series of questionnaires, charts, and forms for you to fill out. Charting symptoms can help to identify triggers and patterns, but it requires nothing more than a pen and a piece of paper, not an expensive diary. (To order from the United States, send $9.95 plus $2.50 postage and handling to Dr. A. H. Goldberg, 920 King Street West, Kitchener, Ontario, Canada N2G 1G4.)

TAPES ON CFS

National and local CFS/CFIDS organizations offer hundreds of audiotapes and videotapes, including overviews of the illness, lectures, and presentations at meetings and conferences. The most widely distributed is Trina Berne's *Chronic Fatigue Syndrome Audiotape*. On the first side of this tape, Berne, a psychotherapist, provides information about CFS and advice about coping with it. She summarizes information about possible causes and some treatments, but makes no commitment to any of the rival hypotheses: "The cause and cure remain unknown." Berne's delineation of the symptoms and dilemmas associated with the illness is straightforward, and her tone is sympathetic, serious, and entirely nonblaming.

The second side of the tape contains a "relaxing and healing" exercise intended, Berne says, not to cure the illness but to serve as an adjunct in treating it. I found the relaxation exercise, as promised, relaxing. Healing? Who knows? (To order, send $9.00 per tape to Trina Berne, M.C., Human Dynamics, 761 East University, Suite A-1, Mesa, Arizona 85203.)

BOOKS ON CHRONIC ILLNESS

I found Cheri Register's *Living with Chronic Illness: Days of Patience and Passion* (1987) to be very helpful. The author has a rare liver disease, and the book is based on her experiences and on interviews with people who had major illnesses. Those people had a broad range of diagnoses, including a seizure disorder, multiple sclerosis, Crohn's disease, and manic depressive illness. Although only one had no diagnosis and no one had chronic fatigue syndrome, this complicated, interesting, realistic book is a must for anyone with a chronic illness. The first chapter, which discusses the whole issue of naming the illness, and the chapter on the etiquette of dealing with chronic illness are, I think, essential reading. *Living with Chronic Illness* is not a self-help guide but an honest, insightful, intelligent discussion of the psychology of chronic illness.

If you want general advice about your illness and your life, words of inspiration, and lists of what to do, the place to look is *We Are Not Alone: Learning to Live the Chronic Illness* (1986) by Sefra K. Pitzele. *We Are Not Alone* spells out the conventional wisdom on accepting your illness. Its aim is not modest: "This is a book about redesigning your life, now that you have a chronic illness. It is a book about how to live better, *not just differently.*"

LIVING WITH CHRONIC FATIGUE

It is so literally a cookbook about illness that it even includes a list of "quick and easy recipes." A great many of the book's nonculinary recipes for living with chronic illnesses were already familiar, such as the advice to rest and to take a positive attitude.

The text is interspersed with inspirational quotations, many of which are the author's quotations of herself.

There are many things about this book that I did not like and many I did not find useful. For example, I really did not find very helpful the glossary that defines *infectious disease specialist* as a doctor who specializes in infectious diseases.

In my negative opinion of *We Are Not Alone*, I am not entirely alone. Leah found it "smarmy." Several people I talked with, however, found the book genuinely helpful and inspirational, and it appears on a number of lists of recommended readings for people with CFS.

The plague in Betty MacDonald's *The Plague and I* (1948) is TB, not CFS, but my former obsession with TB is not the only reason I like this book. MacDonald is best known to adults for *The Egg and I* and best known to children and parents for *Mrs. Piggle-Wiggle* and its various sequels.

In the 1940s, recently divorced and the working mother of young children, Betty MacDonald began to have a series of bad colds. She developed a cough, indigestion, weakness, nervousness, and insomnia. Her tuberculosis was eventually diagnosed, and she was sent to a sanatorium, where she recovered. That potentially maudlin story may not seem to contain the raw ingredients of an entertaining book, but *The Plague and I* is funny, serious, honest, and compassionate. MacDonald offers something rare to anyone with any illness: a model of how to meet it with spirit and without sentimentality.

Minding the Body, Mending the Mind (1987) by Joan Borysenko is based on the work of the Mind Body Program at Boston's Deaconess Hospital. This self-help guide, like the program, emphasizes meditation. Of the dozens of mind-body connection books on the market, this seems the least blaming. It appears here mainly because Roseanne, more willing than the rest of us to believe that she has somehow caused her own illness, calls it "my bible."

MEDICAL GUIDES

The Merck Manual of Diagnosis and Therapy (1982, 1987) is the summary bible of mainstream medicine. Imagine, over 2,500 pages about what might be making you sick! It must be there somewhere. Erik doesn't think so. In fact, he calls the manual "incomplete."

The fourteenth and fifteenth editions are, for the purposes of someone with a chronic fatigue illness, quite similar, and the fourteenth edition may be available at low cost. A major difference is the absence of any reference to AIDS in the fourteenth edition and the presence of plentiful information on it in the fifteenth. Neither edition mentions CFS or CFIDS.

The introduction to the *Manual* says that its primary purpose is "to provide useful information to practicing physicians, medical students, interns, residents, and other health professionals." In other words, it is meant for us only on the principle that every patient becomes his own physician. There is, however, no need to feel guilty about reading it. Almost everyone with a weird illness does.

Most of the *Manual* is a survey of the medical ills of our species. It is organized according to medical specialities: infectious and parasitic disease, immunology and allergic disorders, cardiovascular disorders. After some introductory material, each main section presents chapters on groups of disorders, and each chapter lists the diseases or disorders in its category. Fortunately, in case you don't happen to know the medical category in which you are interested, there is a good index.

At the beginning of the *Manual* is a list of abbreviations and symbols that are absolutely necessary even to begin deciphering the text. Unless you have medical training, you will also need an unabridged dictionary and/or a dictionary of medical terms. Even with the diligent use of a dictionary, a great deal of the *Manual* is incomprehensible to the layperson, and learning what to read and what to ignore is part of learning to use it for your own purposes.

There is, however, a particular risk of using it at all: terror. The *Manual* lists everything you don't want to have, and, particularly

LIVING WITH CHRONIC FATIGUE

if you read it with something less than complete understanding, you may scare yourself into thinking you have something dreadful. The phenomenon of believing that you have what you are reading about is known as Medical Students' syndrome, and it's a disorder that you'd better learn to self-diagnose and treat if you want to consult the *Manual.*

Physicians' Desk Reference, the PDR, is a yearly encyclopedia of information about prescription and nonprescription drugs. Its more than 2,300 pages list more than 2,000 products. The PDR is available in most libraries. If you have any questions about a drug that's been prescribed for you, or any questions about one you've heard has been prescribed for other people, and if your doctor hasn't answered your questions in enough detail to satisfy you, the PDR is the place to look. Of particular importance is the PDR's inclusion of warnings, contraindications, precautions, and adverse reactions.

Much less technical than the PDR, *The Pharmacist's Prescription: Your Complete Guide to the Over-the-Counter Remedies that Work Best* (1987) by F. James Grogan is a sensible guide to remedies that don't work as well as to those that do. It is filled with information: Kaopectate and similar products taste like mud because they contain, you guessed it, mud. None of those over-the-counter remedies is going to cure chronic fatigue syndrome, but if you want to treat symptoms, there are better and worse non-prescription drugs. If the PDR is too much for you, this guide will help you sort them out.

It's Your Body: Know What the Doctor Ordered! (1979) by Marion Fox, R.N., and Truman Schnabel, M.D., is supposed to be a complete guide to medical testing.

The introductory sections are realistic about just how bad an experience diagnostic testing can be. Four case histories presented in the book's first chapter illustrate those points.

After three introductory chapters, the book devotes each of the remaining twelve chapters to diagnostic tests of a particular bodily system. Each of those chapters describes the system and relevant diagnostic tests. The test descriptions take the form of responses to questions: What is the test and why was it ordered? What preparation is needed? How is the test performed? Where is it done and by whom? How much time does it take? How will you feel? Is there a risk?

The explanations of what tests are and why they are performed are comprehensible. So far as I can tell, the estimates of the times the tests take are accurate.

"How will you feel?" means "Is it awful, and, if so, how awful?" This book avoids brutal honesty. To say that a barium enema is "unpleasant" and "not the most dignified of procedures" is to understate many people's pain and embarrassment.

The answers to the question "Is there a risk?" also seem designed more to assure people that risks are minimal than to spell out what the risks really are.

It must be difficult to write a book that informs people about diagnostic testing without scaring them. A book that spells out all the gory details of everything that could ever go wrong will cause unnecessary dread and may even make people refuse necessary tests. This book steers a middle course. If you want to know what a diagnostic test is, this is a useful book, but keep in mind that sometimes "minimal discomfort" may mean "more than minimal."

What You Should Know About Medical Lab Tests (1979) by Bernard Kliman, M.D., and Raymond Vermette, M.S., is a good companion to the *Merck Manual* or *It's Your Body*. Unlike *It's Your Body*, it is almost exclusively about blood and urine tests, and it explains the analyses done on all of those bodily fluids that laboratories examine. The authors succeed in de-mystifying the tests. This is not a book that tells you only that your doctor will understand the tests, but one that actually tells you about them.

The ideal of a doctor-patient partnership is one to which many books pay lip service, but this book contributes to real partnership by sparing doctors the task of giving patients a quick survey course on laboratory medicine and by sparing patients the need to ask for such a course.

CAN LEARNING MORE ABOUT CFS BE HARMFUL?

As I've already confessed, I once read a book about the blood of TB patients. I read it cover to cover. I even studied the tables and charts. Did it help me? Yes and no. Reading that book helped to meet my need to have someone try to figure out what was wrong with me. My effort filled the vacuum left by medicine, but it was an adaptive effort gone sadly awry. In reality, the probability that I had TB was negligible, and even if I had had TB, the book would not have told me so. In retrospect, it is clear to me, if I may paraphrase Leah, that I would have made better use of my limited time and energy if I had pursued something that was part of my regular life, not part of my sickness life. Although I told myself that I was only seeking information, not identity, I was actually letting the illness become central to my identity just when I needed to make it as peripheral as possible. In overdosing on books about illness, I was letting illness become the most important thing in my life.

But, of course, it's easy for me to say that I let illness become too central. I'm healthy. Illness amnesia is probably beginning to set in already. Maybe at the time I really needed to focus on my illness and on TB.

Some people would say, as Alison's internist did, that learning more about CFS will only make a bad situation worse. And maybe I really did let my illness become too central by reading too much. On the whole I suspect that I was a great deal better off for my efforts to learn about CFS. Information can demystify the symptoms, the diagnoses, and the prescriptions and increase your sense of control over the situation. Learning about CFS won't cure you, but it may help you not to feel like its victim.

—10—

Remission and Recovery:

IT DOES HAPPEN

When I was ill, I believed that I would never recover. I was wrong.

"It's now out of my system," Laura says with confidence, and in the three years since her recovery, the illness diagnosed as CEBV has not recurred even when she has missed sleep or felt under stress. Meg has completely recovered from an acute, entirely mysterious illness that was clearly not chronic fatigue syndrome. Ellen and I are no longer ill; we have lingering symptoms. "Sometimes I get that old feeling," says Ginny, "but I rest and feel better." Leah's illness is in remission. Don has relapses from time to time. "Now," says Norma, "I don't feel sick the way I did. Once or twice a week, I'll feel sick. I feel fatigued, and I can't do athletic activities, but I don't feel sick every day."

THE UPS AND DOWNS OF RECOVERY

One day you wake up and realize that your fever has gone. Your glands are not swollen, and nothing hurts. You jump out of bed, run five miles, get your old job back, and take up where you left off.

Sorry, that's not even close. One of the most useful things

my doctor said in the entire course of my illness was something she told me when I broke the news that I was beginning to feel better: recovery from a long illness is not only slow but uneven. Exceptions exist. Laura's recovery was rapid. Nonetheless, for most people, recovery means feeling a little better, then worse, then better, then a little worse, then much better.

Is *recovery* the wrong word? Many people won't use it. I like the word. Maybe I like tempting fate. When I say that I have recovered, do I mean that I am in perfect health and will never again feel ill? Of course not. I have, however, recovered my energy and my sense of physical well-being. I've had a lot of joint pain lately, but it doesn't bother me because I don't feel sick. Is this remission? Maybe life is remission. Does it frighten me to declare that I am well? Yes. Just as it should frighten any other well person. Remember our discussion of the well person's desire to deny illness? Sick people know something well people don't. We have lost the illusion of invulnerability. In a sense, we've grown up in a way they haven't yet.

WHAT WAS THAT NAMELESS FORCE?

A virus? Stress? An immune system dysfunction? Could it have been a familiar, recognized illness that laboratory tests failed to spot? Cytomegalovirus? Toxoplasmosis? Brucellosis? Should some of the tests have been repeated? Would any treatment have cured it? Shortened its course? Made it easier to live with?

When I was ill, I would incorrectly have predicted that recovery would be enough. If only the illness would go away, who'd care what it was? But I still care. There's satisfaction in naming an enemy. A burglar once broke into my house and stole a tape deck, a camera, and my wedding ring. I never found out who the burglar was. He went away, so what does it matter? It's too late to get back what he took. As time passes, I am no longer angry at the burglar, and I care less and less what the illness was, but I remain curious.

TAKING EXTRA CARE

"Today, I run pretty much a normal life on six to seven hours sleep a night," says Greg, but he adds, "I have to be careful." Fully recovered, Laura still says: "I'm very careful." Although I suspect that I am careless compared to most people who have recovered or who have improved greatly, I am, by any ordinary standards, very careful, too. What does careful mean? Getting a lot of sleep, eating right, and, for many people, following whatever program helped. Are we paranoid or compulsive? No, we just scare easily. Fatigue panics us. Why? Because we're not naive any more.

THE PSYCHOLOGICAL AFTERMATH

One of the discouraging and surprising features of becoming ill is to find yourself defeated in just those areas in which you had previously sensed yourself to be especially competent. In eroding physical, emotional, intellectual, social, and vocational abilities, this illness provides a solid basis for perceptions of inadequacy. It challenges your ability to feel competent in the face of mounting evidence of failure.

I know as I never did before how weak, incompetent, lethargic, muddle-headed, and selfish I can become. I know how it feels to try my best and fail badly. My own work does not conquer all. I cannot rely on myself to think my way out of trouble. If times really get tough, they may just stay tough. In some fundamental way, my world is less predictable and trustworthy than it used to be.

For me, physical recovery alone left a painful psychological aftermath of mistrust, shame and doubt, guilt, and all the rest. Only in letting myself hear the people I've called Alex, Alison, Andy, Don, Ellen, Erik, Ginny, and all of the others did I really recover.

REASON TO HOPE

The loss of psychological vitality that accompanies illness provides an unlikely basis for a healthy self-image and a likely one for despair. I don't claim to be able to recognize a healthy self-image—but I know what despair is. And I heard surprisingly little during the course of my interviews. In retrospect, I realize that I was originally afraid to hear people talk about their illnesses; indeed, I had avoided other ill people during my own illness because I expected a mirror of my own despair. I was afraid to hear people say that they had put their lives on hold. I did hear sadness, impatience, and anger, especially anger at the illness and anger at responses to it. But I also heard strength and vitality. I even heard Wendy say that she was happy despite her sickness.

Despite the difficulties of having the illness—the stress in dealing with the medical profession, the strain on interpersonal relationships, and the problems you may encounter in the workplace—there's reason to be hopeful. So many of the people with whom I've talked have found ways to cope with this baffling illness and get on with their lives. I hope that you can, too.

References

Berkow, Robert, ed. *The Merck Manual of Diagnosis and Therapy*. 15th ed. Rahway, N.J.: Merck and Company, 1987.

Berne, Trina. *Chronic Fatigue Syndrome Audiotape*. Mesa, Ariz.: Human Dynamics.

Borysenko, Joan, with Larry Rothstein. *Minding the Body, Mending the Mind*. New York: Bantam Books, 1987.

Brooks, Barbara, and Nancy Smith. *CFIDS: An Owner's Manual*. Silver Spring, Md.: BBNS, 1988.

Cheney, Paul R., M.D., Ph.D. Statement to the Senate Appropriations Subcommittee on Labor, Health and Human Services, and Education. 8 May 1989. *CFIDS Chronicle* (Spring 1989).

"Chronic Fatigue Syndrome." *Harvard Medical School Health Letter* 13 (July 1988).

Crook, William G. *The Yeast Connection*. New York: Vintage Books, 1987.

Endsley, John W. *Understanding Chronic Fatigue Syndrome: Practical Information for Patients*.

Fisher, Gregg Charles, and Stephen E. Straus, M.D., Paul R. Cheney, M.D., Ph.D., and James M. Oleske, M.D. *Chronic Fatigue Syndrome*. New York: Warner Books, 1989.

Fisher, Gregg Charles, and Caren Heacock, Bernard Fisher, Stephen E. Straus, M.D., and James Oleske, M.D. *Waiting to Live: The Debilitating Effects of Chronic Epstein-Barr Virus*. Upper Montclair, N.J.: Montco, 1987.

Friedlander, Mark P. and Terry M. Phillips. *Winning the War Within: Understanding, Protecting, and Building Your Body's Immunity.* Emmaus, Pa.: Rodale Press, 1986.

Fox, Marion L., and Truman G. Schnabel. *It's Your Body: Know What The Doctor Ordered! Your Complete Guide to Medical Testing.* Bowie, Md.: The Charles Press, 1979.

Goldberg, Arnold H., M.D. *Chronic Fatigue Syndrome: A Personal Diary.* Kitchener, Ontario, Canada: Alexarn Associates Ltd., 1988.

Grogan, James F. *The Pharmacist's Prescription: Your Complete Guide to the Over-the-Counter Remedies That Work Best.* New York: Rawson Associates, 1987.

Holmes, G. P., and J. E. Kaplan, N. M. Gantz, A. L. Komaroff, L. B. Schonberger, S. E. Straus, J. F. Jones, R. E. Dubois, C. Cunningham-Rundles, S. Pahwa, G. Tosato, L. S. Zegans, D. T. Purtilo, N. Brown, R. T. Schooley, and I. Brus. "Chronic Fatigue Syndrome: A Working Case Definition." *Annals of Internal Medicine* 108 (March 1988).

Houston CFIDS Support Group. *Chronic Fatigue and Immune Dysfunction (Chronic Epstein-Barr Virus) Syndrome: Patient Information.* 4th ed. Houston, Tex. (Available through The Houston CFIDS Support Group, 8820 Memorial Drive, Houston, TX 77024.)

Iverson, Marc M. "In Response to Mr. Edelson." *CFIDS Chronicle* (Spring 1989).

Johnson, Hillary. "Journey Into Fear: The Growing Nightmare of Epstein-Barr Virus." *Rolling Stone* 504/505 (16 July 1987) and 506 (13 August 1987).

Kliman, Bernard, and Raymond Vermette with Ernest Kolowrat. *What You Should Know About Medical Lab Tests.* New York: Thomas Y. Crowell, Publishers, 1979.

Light, Richard J., and David Pillemer. *Summing Up: The Science of Reviewing Research.* Cambridge, Mass. and London: Harvard University Press, 1984.

MacDonald, Betty. *The Plague and I.* Philadelphia and New York: J. B. Lippincott, 1948.

Physicians' Desk Reference. 42nd ed. Oradell, N.J.: Medical Economics Company, Inc., Edward R. Barnhart, Publisher, 1988.

Pitzele, Sefra K. *We Are Not Alone: Learning to Live with Chronic Illness.* New York: Workman Publishing, 1986.

Register, Cheri. *Living with Chronic Illness: Days of Patience and Passion.* New York: The Free Press, 1987.

Stoff, Jesse A., M.D. and Charles Pellegrino, Ph.D. *Chronic Fatigue Syndrome: The Hidden Epidemic.* New York: Random House, 1988.

Straus, Stephen E. "The Chronic Mononucleosis Syndrome." *Journal of Infectious Disease* 157 (1988).

Thomson, Dick. "Stealthy Epidemic of Exhaustion: Doctors Are Perplexed by the Mysterious 'Yuppie Disease.'" Reported by Scott Brown and Steven Holmes. *Time* 29 June 1987.

Van Zelst, Theodore W. Statement to the House Appropriations Subcommittee on Labor, Health and Human Services, and Education. 1 May 1989. *CFIDS Chronicle* (Spring 1989).

"Yeast: Raising Questions." *Harvard Medical School Health Letter* 12 (February 1987).